BREAD
THERAPY

BREAD
THERAPY

THE MINDFUL ART
OF BAKING BREAD

PAULINE BEAUMONT

Houghton Mifflin Harcourt

Boston • New York • 2020

For information about permission to reproduce selections
from this book, write to trade.permissions@hmhco.com or to
Permissions, Houghton Mifflin Harcourt Publishing Company,
3 Park Avenue, 19th Floor, New York, New York 10016.

hmhbooks.com

Library of Congress Cataloging-in-Publication Data is available.

ISBN 978-0-358-51903-4

Illustrations © Shutterstock.com

Book design by Briony Hartley

Printed in the United States of America

DOC 10 9 8 7 6 5 4 3 2 1

Dedicated to Sarah, Becky, Jonny,
Thomas, Violet, and Rose

About the Author

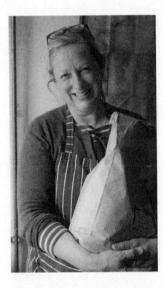

After studying Psychology and Philosophy, Pauline Beaumont began a 20-year career in the arts. A return to higher education led to a new career in mental health and her current work as a student counselor at her old university.

Big families have figured largely in her life. She is the oldest of six siblings and has six, now grown up, children herself. While bringing up her family and working in the north of England, baking bread became increasingly important to her. She found the pattern of breadmaking shaped her days, as it continues to do, providing an antidote to the inevitable stresses of life.

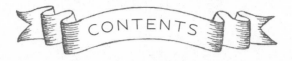

CONTENTS

Introduction

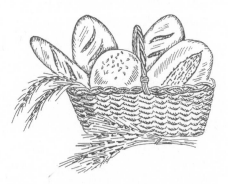

For many of us, time can feel like a scarce commodity. Like Lewis Carroll's White Rabbit, we charge around, fearing we will be late and worrying about fitting everything in. Why, you might ask, would we want to add baking bread to our already lengthy to-do list?

This book answers that question. Making time to bake your own bread will help you to reap many rewards. The more frenetic our lives, the more we need the balance that comes from activities that force us to slow down and reconnect us to our physicality. Making our own bread gives us these soothing and grounding experiences in spades. "Making time" is a fascinating and helpful concept. While, of course, we can't create more time than the

24 hours each day offers us, we can choose to pause, to build into our days precious periods of focus and mindfulness that serve as an antidote to the pressures of our otherwise fast-paced lives. I have found that making bread provides me with just such a regular dose of unhurried, creative activity that is joyful, calming, and productive. I want to show you all the ways in which making your own bread could enrich your life, too, and inspire you to delight in, and benefit from, getting your hands into some dough.

There is something about the metamorphosis of flour and water into a loaf of bread that is entrancing and that always feels a little miraculous. The realization that—with your own hands—you can make something so delicious and nutritious from scratch is a revelation and easier to achieve than you might think. Once you can bake your own bread, you know that you will always be able to produce nourishing loaves for your family from pantry ingredients.

But the magic of breadmaking is much more than this. The process of going back to primal principles, of working with basic ingredients, provides us with an opportunity to learn and to be 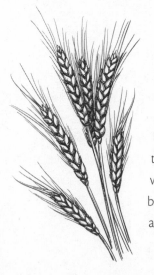 creative in ways that can have a lasting, positive impact on our well-being. I often think that there are parallels between being a breadmaker and being a potter—mixing dough or clay, forming loaves or pots, and waiting to see what emerges from the oven or kiln. Like becoming a potter, to become a breadmaker is to become a craftsperson. It is something that will enrich your life as well as your larder and can become part of your identity—part of who you are as well as what you do.

I sometimes lose track of time when I'm baking bread, and it reminds me of how, as a child, I would lose myself in reading. An early literary memory is the description of bread in Johanna Spyri's *Heidi*. I was fascinated by the hard black bread and the cheese wrapped in a cloth that Heidi was given to eat by her grandfather in their mountain hut and then the soft, white rolls she loved at Fräulein Rottenmeier's townhouse. I remember being in awe of her self-sacrifice in giving up the pleasure of eating the delicious bread to save the rolls for Peter the goatherd's grandmother back home. My perspective would be different now and my adult self would yell at Heidi, "Eat the bread!"

Growing up, my grandfather didn't live in the Alps, but in Sunderland, and my parents, my five siblings, and I would visit him for tea every Sunday. He used to buy us each a miniature Hovis loaf—they were about 3 inches long with the logo raised on the side. I loved each little loaf; the desire to preserve its wholeness pitted against the urge to cut it into tiny slices and wolf it down. Brown bread was a bit of a rarity for us. It would be neat to be able to tell you about my mother imparting the joy of breadmaking to me in clouds of flour and affection, but she did not bake bread. She bought Mother's Pride sliced white bread and I loved that too.

I came to breadmaking fairly late in life and I see this, at least partly, as being the result of a 1970s, girls' school, polarized take on feminism. The choice seemed to be between Simone de Beauvoir and *The Stepford Wives*. This meant that anything to do with household tasks had to be shunned at all costs to avoid the dreaded fate of ending up as some sort of domestic slave. It took me a long time to realize that baking bread and freedom of choice were compatible. I moved gradually from a resigned obligation to feed my family to a realization that I actually enjoyed messing around in the kitchen for hours and time would fly in the same way as it did when I was lost in a book. Baking bread started to take a central role in my cooking and, on the eve of a day off work, I would fall asleep thinking about what sort of bread I might start making in the morning. If I had some dough rising, I might sneak downstairs to have a look at it in the middle of the night. I hope that this excitement in making bread never leaves me, and that this book might help you to find it too.

In parts of the world where people struggle to feed themselves (or at times in our own history), making bread has constituted an unavoidable part of the daily grind rather than a source of pleasure and fulfillment. However, it does seem that the more that digital and remote ways of interacting dominate our lives, the more we appreciate the opposite; the benefits of a return to basics, the natural, the handmade, and the real. We recognize the merits of walking, even though we could get to our destination more quickly by car; we relish the joys of growing our own vegetables, despite the labors involved; and we might sometimes spend days knitting a sweater, rather than buying one from a shop. This book is about the value of making bread by hand, from choice rather than necessity, and the benefits that can result for our health and well-being.

Bread Therapy is a kneading together of seven factors that contribute to emotional and psychological well-being. It describes how baking bread can provide us with the ingredients for a fulfilled life. In my work as a therapist, I am constantly faced with the damaging impact of perfectionism on mental health. Accepting that nothing is perfect and that we all make mistakes is therefore highly beneficial. There are lots of things that can, and often do, go wrong when we are baking bread, so it provides us with lots of opportunities to practice accepting the imperfect. This acceptance of imperfection, and in turn our own fallibility, is a stepping stone to developing greater self-compassion and improved psychological well-being.

Being able to bake our own bread affords us increased self-sufficiency in difficult times. Understanding ourselves better and learning about the different ways we can support our mental health, as described in this book, also puts us in a position to take more responsibility for our own well-being. *Bread Therapy* will show you how, through learning to make your own bread, you can also learn essential life lessons.

I have a passion for making bread, and I want you to benefit from this craft that unites people all over the world and also links us with our ancestors. Bread has a universal, symbolic resonance: It is a metaphor for transformation, the bringing together of unprepossessing ingredients into something that is glorious. Making bread can be a reminder to us all that we, too, are capable of transformation.

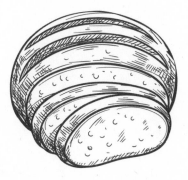

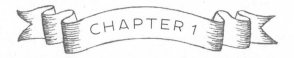

CHAPTER 1

Being Physical

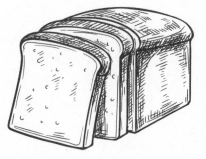

HANDMADE

For me, a feeling of deep contentment comes early in the morning when I am not at work and the house is full. As my family sleeps, I'll come downstairs to meet a small row of baking pans or baskets of risen dough. I'll make coffee as the oven heats up, and before long, the air is full of the soothing smell of baking bread. By the time sleepy faces appear at the kitchen door, the dough has been transformed into golden sourdough or nutty brown loaves of spelt or rye on the cooling rack, and breakfast begins.

There seems to be an atavistic pleasure in making something with your own hands and then giving it to others. The making of food and the feeding of people around us is a profound example of this and the baking and sharing of bread is fundamental to our humanity and our connectedness. The word "companion" comes from the Latin words for "with" (*com*) and for "bread" (*panis*). The word was used to describe a person you shared food with. We now use the word companion in a wider sense to mean a friend, someone who goes alongside us. The ritual of baking bread has become a companion to me; an activity that punctuates my weeks, bonds me with others, and connects me with my own physicality.

Think about ordering your groceries online and picture clicking on a plastic-wrapped, mass-manufactured loaf of sliced bread. Then, in comparison, imagine yourself kneading a fragrant lump of dough you have made from local, stone-ground flour, waiting for it to rise, and then continuing the ritual until you have a freshly baked, delicious, and nourishing loaf or two.

The first version of acquiring bread is undoubtedly quicker and cheaper, but there is something in the—admittedly—laborious nature of the breadmaking process, the handling of ingredients, the harnessing of time and heat, that has value as an aid to good mental health, in addition to producing an infinitely better loaf of bread. Making bread is good for the body, the mind and, some would say, the soul. One of the ways that making bread is good for us is through giving us an opportunity to reconnect with our physicality, to exert ourselves, to use our hands and at the same time be mindful of every sensory aspect of the activity.

The baking and sharing of bread is fundamental to our humanity and our connectedness.

Freud extolled the merits of work and love as the key compon-
ents of a good life. Making bread by hand is both hard work and
can be thought of as a labor of love. We don't have to do it, so if
we choose to, then maybe we are indeed doing it for the love of
the process as well as the product. In the same way that tending
a garden to grow our own vegetables is not the easiest way of
getting our hands on a pound of green beans, so it is with making
our own bread.

The idea that there is something redeeming and spiritual about
simple, physical work is not necessary for us to benefit from the
activity, but from George Herbert's notion of divine drudgery to
the Buddhist idea of doing chores as a spiritual practice, there is
a long tradition of achieving some sort of transcendence through
the routine and the mundane. Making bread by hand falls into this
category. Becoming absorbed in the physicality of the experience
of making bread can become a meditation in itself. Making bread is
a simple way to build a mind-body connection.

HEALTH IN MIND AND BODY

The appreciation that physical activity is beneficial for mental as
well as physical health is now a well-established tenet of contemporary Western medicine. The benefits of understanding health
in a holistic way are nothing new to many cultures and medical
traditions and, belatedly, Western medicine has started to catch
up. There is now recognition that the reality is that it is impossible
to separate the mind from the body. There is an acknowledgment
that what we do with our bodies will have a profound impact on

Engaging in physical activity — touching materials, moving and making things — can have a positive impact on how well we feel emotionally.

our emotional and mental health. Conversely, it is very hard to feel mentally well if you are not eating well, not sleeping well, and not exercising or moving enough. It is this good-enough mental well-being which is exemplified in a reasonably positive sense of ourselves, other people, the world, and the future.

It is a strange paradox that living too much in our heads can be bad for our mental health, while engaging in physical activity—touching materials, moving, and making things—can have a positive impact on how well we feel emotionally.

THE PHYSICAL ACTIVITY OF KNEADING

Baking your own bread might not be the most strenuous form of exercise, but what it does present us with is a physical activity that is grounding and that can be alternately soothing or energizing. It provides us with a way of connecting with our senses and using our hands. It is translating our own muscle power and the energy we put into the process into a beautiful and nourishing end result.

To knead is to variously work and press and pull the dough into a smooth mixture with the hands. Kneading is hard work, repetitive, and it is real. There is no virtual or digital equivalent of making your own bread by hand. Using a breadmaking machine can produce decent bread, but I would argue that it is the process as much as the product that gives making bread by hand such a satisfying and potentially therapeutic quality. There is no substitute for getting your fingers sticky with dough and even aching with the sustained effort of thorough kneading. Kneading your bread dough will involve muscles in your fingers, hands, wrists, arms, shoulders, and even your back that you might not usually use. You will know this is the case because, as you start to develop your own style of kneading, you may feel tiredness and soreness exactly as you would after other sorts of physical exertion.

Kneading bread dough is a wonderful example of a skill that we can grow and improve over time. Looking online or in books will soon show you that there is no one, right way of doing it. Making bread is an art as much as a science. As well as personal preference, there are many variables that will influence how much or what sort of kneading works best.

WHY DO WE KNEAD?

The purpose of kneading—or working the dough—is to make sure that all the ingredients are evenly mixed, and to develop gluten. Gluten is a mixture of proteins including glutenin and gliadin. It is important for breadmaking as it allows for a stretchiness in the dough, which means that gases produced in the rising process can be held in the dough and then allow the bread to expand and rise. Gluten development is a chemical process that begins when the dough is mixed and is enhanced by kneading. Long strands of protein molecules are formed that create a network of strands which, in turn, give bread its structure.

There are some breads, such as soda breads, whose rapid rise is created by the reaction between baking soda and the acid in buttermilk, and these doughs need no kneading. At the other end of the time spectrum, the lengthy fermentation process that characterizes deeply flavored sourdough bread means that the desired texture can develop with much less working than a yeasted dough would require. Another variable is the flour you are using. Different flours have differing amounts and types of gluten. For example, rye flour is low in gluten, so it will not benefit from much kneading.

There are many kneading methods. Try them, combine them, change them, and develop your own way of working the dough to achieve the desired, smooth, silky, and bouncy dough that will result in a loaf that can hold its shape and rise well in the oven.

All kneading methods involve mixing and then working the ingredients for your dough using your fingers, your knuckles, the heel of your hands, or your fists with as much energy as you can manage for at least 10 minutes. You can pull, push, stretch, pummel, fold, turn, and squash the dough. It is sometimes necessary to get our hands very sticky when kneading, which might feel uncomfortable; we are not used to it and often feel driven to add more flour in the early stages, before the existing flour has had a chance to absorb all of the water in the mix. Accept the stickiness, keep going. As a general rule, the wetter the dough, the better the bread.

If you watch expert bakers kneading, you will see wonderful variations involving holding the dough up in the air while working it or slapping it down on the work surface in a way that incorporates more air, which lightens the dough.

Experiment, and whichever way of working the dough becomes your signature style, there is the potential to use this intense period of physical activity as a focus for the potent, parallel activity of mindfulness.

MINDFUL BAKING

For all of us, there is no escaping from stress, but there are ways we can help ourselves to become more resilient and to be able to cope better with inevitable challenges. Mindfulness is a powerful way of improving our capacity to cope with stress and with anxiety and depression. At its most simple level, mindfulness involves us paying more attention to the present, to the moment we are in now. It involves us placing our attention, deliberately, on our own thoughts, feelings, or senses and the world around us in a quiet and dispassionate way. By concentrating on our senses, what we can hear, see, smell, touch, feel, and taste, we can connect better with our bodies and our physical nature. We can slow down and put our attention away from ourselves and our rushing thoughts. By putting our attention on what we are thinking, feeling, and sensing, we remind ourselves that we are not our thoughts or feelings; there is a part of us that can observe them and let them go by. This ability to shift our minds into observer mode is a valuable tool in fostering mental well-being.

Ten or fifteen minutes of kneading bread dough can provide a rare opportunity to concentrate on one thing at a time. While we may be exerting ourselves physically as we knead, mindfulness—in this case the practice of moving our attention away from our racing thoughts and placing it on our senses—is a form of meditation. To knead dough mindfully is a way of slowing down, of giving ourselves the opportunity to be present in the moment, to be aware of the feel of the sticky dough on our hands, to recognize the change in the feel of the dough as it develops, to smell the yeast, to see the appearance of the dough's surface alter, and to hear the sounds of the dough peeling off the work surface and the hum of the warming oven.

> To knead dough mindfully is a way of slowing down, of giving ourselves the opportunity to be present in the moment.

It has become normal for many of us to do lots of things at the same time, for example cooking while watching TV or glancing back and forth at a computer screen. We might be walking while talking on the phone or running while listening to music on headphones. This layering of activity is so usual that it can be quite disconcerting to give all of our attention to one thing at a time. When we have become habituated to being overstimulated, then quietness, stillness, slowing down, and having a single focus can feel awkward at first. For many of us, activity can be a way of masking anxiety. Paradoxically, when we start to slow down, this can temporarily present us with a new challenge of having to face the feeling of anxiety. Daring to turn off the cacophony of content from our phones and screens may cause us to feel initial unease, but adapting ourselves to increasing stillness and focus on our senses—

becoming more mindful—can provide us with a sustainable way of managing anxiety for the rest of our lives.

The physical process of breadmaking provides us with an ideal opportunity to develop mindfulness skills, which can then have far-reaching benefits for our mental well-being.

As you gather the ingredients and equipment to bake, concentrate on what you can see, hear, feel, and smell. Feel the weight and smoothness of your mixing bowl. Let the flour run through your fingers and try to detect its subtle scent. Test the temperature of the water with your fingers. As you slowly mix the flour and water and yeast, feel the changing textures, the stickiness, and then the developing smoothness and stretchiness of the dough. How does it smell now? How does the surface of the dough look?

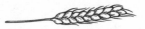

Learning to be more mindful is one of the most important skills you can develop. If we are being mindful, then we naturally slow down and become calmer and more relaxed, but the true value of practicing mindfulness lies in it being a way of training our attention. If we are focused on our senses then, as we can only really focus on one thing at a time, we will be less likely to be thinking worrying thoughts. Our attention is one of the most precious commodities we possess and one of the least appreciated. It is easily squandered or stolen—for example, our attention is the commodity capitalized on by social media companies that knowingly entice us to spend increasing chunks of our time on their sites. Common mental health problems such as anxiety and depression, in their many forms, are also voracious thieves of your attention. The tendency to become anxious and worry excessively will mean that attention is often monopolized by negative thoughts about past events or hypothetical disasters, "Why did I say that?" or "What if I get sick?" And the pessimistic mindset that characterizes both depression and low self-esteem means that your attention will be preferentially pulled to evidence that supports a negative view of yourself and the world.

For example, if there is one unsmiling face in your group of friends when you have told them something funny, that is the face you will focus on and you will use it to confirm your (distorted) view that you are not funny or that people don't like you. This is the result of a powerful combination of selective attention and confirmation bias. Selective attention is a necessary filtering of all of the information we are constantly bombarded with. We need the focus it provides, but the way our minds select the object for our attention is influenced by confirmation bias. This is the tendency we have to see and hear things that confirm what we already believe, such as the belief that one is not liked being confirmed by seeing the one unsmiling face. We focus on certain material that tends to confirm what we already believe and filter out any contradictory evidence. When we are depressed or have low self-esteem, then we believe that the world is a disappointing and dreadful place and that we are not good enough. An evening out with friends that involves hours of relaxed conversation and laughter might be followed by days of rumination over one ill-timed joke that did not go down well. So attention is disproportionately focused on the single, perceived, negative element of the evening rather than seeing the positive whole. This attentional bias then further confirms negative beliefs such as "I'm no good socially" or "People will think I'm stupid."

Worrying will not help in any of these situations, but it is highly seductive, and some might say addictive; it is so habit-forming. Worrying excessively is a habit we can break, and mindfulness is one of the tools we can use to do this. Developing the ability to divert our attention from one thing to another, through mindfulness, allows us to shift attention from an unhelpful, self-critical, or catastrophizing thought to something we actually want or need to be concentrating on.

Practicing mindfulness by treating breadmaking as a form of meditation—paying attention to what we can sense and what we are doing physically throughout the process—allows us to hone our ability to take charge of our attention. It is similar to the way in which we physically train our muscles through repeating an exercise. By using breadmaking as the focal "exercise," we can practice pulling our attention back to our senses. As our mind inevitably wanders, we can get better and better at noticing this and returning our attention to our dough. This skill is central to our ability to manage our own emotional state and psychological well-being.

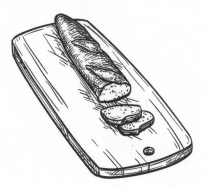

A MINDFUL LOAF

It's time to make your first mindful loaf of bread. Feel the cool heaviness as you press the dough into the oiled and floured pan. Be aware of the time passing as the dough slowly expands in the warmth of the kitchen air. Hear the sounds of the oven. See the changing shape as the dough reaches the top of the pan and is ready to bake. Notice how the smell changes as the baking progresses and the yeasty, dough smell shifts into the sweet aroma of caramelizing crust. Feel the wave of heat as you open the oven. Hear the hollowness as you knock the base of the loaf that tells you it is done. As your loaf sits on the cooling rack, listen carefully for the "song of bread"—the tiny sounds bakers say they can hear from the crust as the bread cools down.

It is normal when we are doing something for the first time to feel unsure and incompetent. The only way to become more adept at any skill is to keep going, to practice, to persevere. If you haven't baked a loaf of bread before, the following recipe for making a yeasted loaf is a wonderfully simple way to start. Allow yourself to feel unsure and unconfident; don't judge yourself, it is fine to feel like that. If you are a more seasoned baker, try making a loaf "as if" you are doing it for the first time. Slow down and focus on the sights, smells, sounds, and feel of what you are doing.

Equipment and ingredients

Start by gathering the equipment and ingredients you need to make your mindful bread.

Essential starting points are access to an oven, a clean work surface, and time. It may only take you 20 minutes to mix and knead your dough, but then you will have up to 2 hours to wait as the yeasted dough rises. Your bread will take another 30–40 minutes to bake and then at least another 30 minutes to cool down. Regard this time as a gift and think what you'll do with it. Perhaps resist the temptation to check your phone or laptop and continue with a mindful approach—give your attention completely to playing with your children, go for a walk, or read a book.

If baking your own bread becomes a part of your everyday life, then you may well delight in collecting breadmaking paraphernalia, such as proofing baskets, scrapers, cooling racks, and myriad pans. But to start with, all you'll need is a large mixing bowl, a measuring cup, a kitchen scale, a loaf pan or baking sheet, and a cooling rack. Choose a loaf pan that is approximately 6 cups in volume, which is roughly 8½ x 4½ x 2½ inches. If you don't have them, for this recipe you could do without the scale or measuring cup by using half of a 2-lb bag of flour and a mug of water. For the flour, it is worth paying more for stone-ground flour, both for taste and nutritional value (see page 59).

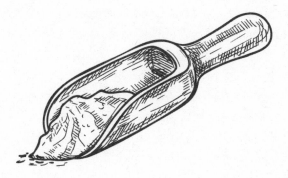

A simple yeasted loaf

Throughout the process, your mind will wander and thoughts of tomorrow or yesterday will flit into your consciousness. Recognize and accept the thoughts and choose not to go with them, but to take your attention back to what you are doing. Focus on your hands, the dough, the sounds, and smells of baking bread.

You can either bake your loaf in a loaf pan or you can bake it free-form on a lined baking sheet. The pan has the advantage of supporting the dough as it rises, producing an oblong loaf with good depth. A disadvantage is that the loaf can sometimes stick, although thorough oiling and flouring the inside of the pan should prevent this.

A free-form loaf is round or oval in shape and will have a lovely crust over a bigger area than the pan loaf. It will never stick on the lined baking sheet, but a disadvantage can be that you can sometimes end up with a rather flat loaf if the dough spreads out too much.

The addition of oil produces a softer crumb and lengthens the time you will be able to keep the loaf, but is not essential.

Makes 1 loaf

INGREDIENTS

oil, for greasing

4¼ cups (18 oz/500 g) white bread flour, plus extra for the
   pan and for dusting

1 tsp fine salt (unrefined sea salt if possible, as this has
   more mineral content than table salt)

1 envelope (2¼ tsp/7 g) fast-acting yeast

1 tsp sugar (optional; sugar can speed up the rising
   process and add to the browning of the crust through
   caramelization)

2 tbsp oil (optional; I use cold-pressed canola oil because
   it has a very mild flavor)

1¼ cups (300 ml) warm water

METHOD

1. Prepare your loaf pan by wiping it thoroughly inside
   with some oil on a paper towel. Then shake some flour
   into the pan and turn it around until there is a thin
   coating all over. Alternatively, if you are making a free-form
   loaf, cover a baking sheet with baking parchment.

2. In a large bowl, mix together the flour, salt, and yeast
   (and sugar, if you are using it).

3. If you are using oil, add it to the warm water (the
   temperature should be such that when you put your

fingers into the water, it doesn't feel hot or cold), and then add the liquid to the dry ingredients, mixing at first with a spoon and then start to use your hands.

4. Begin the kneading in the bowl until the dough is holding together, then continue to knead on a lightly floured work surface for 10 minutes.

5. Your dough is now ready for its first rise. Place it back in the bowl and cover the bowl with a damp dish towel. This is to protect the dough and stop it from drying out. The cloth needs to cover the top of the bowl without touching the dough—I find fixing it over the bowl with two clothespins works well. Leave the ball of dough in a warm place until it has doubled in size. This will take between 30 minutes and an hour depending on how warm your kitchen is.

6. The next stage is called "knocking back." Give your dough a bit of a pummeling to knock out some of the air and you are ready to shape your dough for its second rise.

7. Shape the dough to a size that fits your pan with any seams underneath and a smooth surface on top. Alternatively, to make a more "free-form" loaf, place the dough, shaped into a round, on the lined baking sheet.

8. Your dough now needs time to rise a second time. Cover it with a clean, damp dish towel and leave it in a warm place (your kitchen counter at normal

room temperature is fine), until it has doubled in size. Depending on the temperature and other variables, this will take up to an hour.

9. Heat the oven to 450°F/230°C so that it is up to temperature when the dough is fully risen.

10. Remove the damp cloth and bake the loaf in the center of the oven for approximately 35 minutes.

11. Ovens vary and you will need to use your eyes and nose to judge when it is time to take the bread out of the oven. When your bread is a golden-brown color and you can smell the wonderful aroma of freshly baked bread, which is hard to describe but unmistakable when you smell it, then your loaf is probably done. Remove it from the oven and, in the case of a loaf pan, bang the pan hard on the work top (this is to loosen the bread from the pan) and leave for a minute before turning out the loaf. If the loaf does not come out of the pan right away when you turn it over and shake it, then you will need to carefully run a knife between the bread and the pan. You won't have this problem with a loaf on a baking sheet, but without the support of the pan sides you will have a flatter loaf. Hold the loaf with a cloth and knock your knuckles on its underside. If the loaf is done, it will sound hollow. If you think the bread needs a few more minutes of baking, then put the loaf straight back onto the oven rack. You can also do this to crisp up or brown

the sides of the loaf that have been protected by the pan.

12. Once ready, place your loaf on a cooling rack. As the bread cools it produces steam, which needs to evaporate; the cooling rack is made of wire mesh, which allows the air to circulate all around. If your loaf is on a solid surface, then this steam has nowhere to go and could produce sogginess. If you don't have a cooling rack, you could improvise by using a (cold) oven rack. or the rack from a roasting pan.

13. Overcoming the temptation to eat hot bread straight from the oven requires willpower and will be rewarded by bread in which the starch has developed fully, and the steam has been reabsorbed into the crumb. If you cut into bread when it is still warm, you risk it being a bit soggy. The crumb or texture of your bread will go on becoming firmer and more defined as the loaf cools. This makes it easier to slice.

14. Enjoy your homemade loaf.

Having mindfully made your own bread, you can now eat it mindfully too. Bite and chew it slowly, savoring the taste and smell and feel of it. We so often take the physical process of eating for granted, so be aware of it and slow down; enjoy every mouthful. Take a moment to appreciate the bread you have made yourself by hand.

I have been making bread for over 10 years now and the sense of expectation and pleasure that comes from taking a loaf out of the oven is the same now as it was when I started. I hope you feel this too.

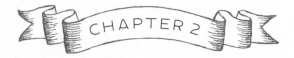

Nurture

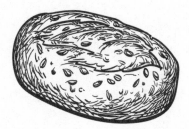

DON'T FEED THE DUCKS

There is a notice by the edge of many lakes in public parks that speaks volumes about the quality of some of the food we put into our mouths. These lakes are often home to swans and ducks. The signs ask that the public refrain from feeding the birds white bread, because it makes them ill and sometimes kills them. The birds usually forage for aquatic weeds, seeds, worms, insects, and small crustaceans, which all provide them with the various nutrients they rely on for healthy development. If they fill up on white bread, which does not provide the nutrients they need, then they do not eat the natural food found in and around the lake and they get sick. Manufactured white bread is not good for birds. It is not good for people, either, but millions of these white, sliced, processed loaves are sold in supermarkets every day (without any health warnings). Not all bread is equal. The difference between white factory-made bread and loaves baked from whole-grain, stone-ground, organic flour is like the difference between chalk and cheese. Actually, chalk (calcium carbonate) used to be outlawed as an adulterant of flour but is now allowed as an additive. One of the best ways of ensuring that the bread you and your family eat is nutritious and is a positive contributor to your health is to bake it yourself with ingredients you have chosen.

I think one of the simplest ways to set about improving our diets is to start from where we are and, one thing at a time, start making healthier substitutions. We might drink water instead of sweetened drinks, we might start using whole-grain pasta and rice instead of their refined versions. If we start making our own nutritious bread then we can achieve the win-win of avoiding the "ducks in the park" scenario. We can avoid filling up on the empty calories of processed bread that actively damage our health, and include something in our diet which will make a significant and positive contribution to our well-being.

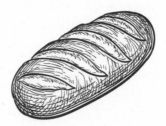

BROWN, WHITE, BROWN

It used to be customary to make your own bread or buy it from a small baker who used traditional methods. However, this became more unusual as mass-produced and supermarket bread became the norm. Now, as an understanding of and interest in healthy eating grows, there is a welcome resurgence of home breadmaking and an appreciation of high-quality loaves made by artisan and small bakeries. Issues of cost and capacity and the scale of demand make a return to complete reliance on small bakeries unlikely, but there is no limit to the number of us who could be taking real breadmaking back into our homes and hearths.

The history of breadmaking is as full of twists and turns as a pretzel. The first evidence of grains being cultivated for breadmaking comes from Egypt in the third millennium BC, but there are signs that wild wheat and barley were being harvested long before this. The practice of grinding grain to make flour and the making of leavened or unleavened bread either at home or in small bakeries developed across the globe. In the West, this pattern of production remained the norm and was regulated from the thirteenth century until the time of the Industrial Revolution. As the population moved to towns and cities for work, a proliferation of bakeries opened. Competition between them increased, rules were ignored, and adulteration of flour to improve profits became widespread. Writing in *The English Bread Book* in 1857, the early cookery writer Eliza Acton bemoaned the declining nutritional value of bread bought from bakers and the unhealthy addition of chemicals such as alum to bulk out ingredients. Most bread at this time was still whole-wheat, as before 1870 there was only stone-ground wheat, which meant that white flour (or whiteish flour) was a bit of a rarity. At the time, white flour was made by sifting out the bran, which was a labor-intensive process, hence the high cost. This increased cost of producing white flour meant that it was mostly the preserve of the wealthy.

By 1880, across Europe and America, metal rollers in mills were introduced. These rollers meant that not only the bran but also the wheat germ were removed from the grain in the milling process and the first "refined" flour was produced. White flour had now become the cheapest flour to produce. The removal of the bran and wheat germ from the whole grain resulted in a reduction in the nutritional value of the flour, but it made good business sense as it produced flour that lasted much longer. Through the twentieth century, milling became increasingly industrialized and, using fast-moving metal rollers, the heat produced in the process of milling further degraded any nutrients left in the flour.

This industrialization of the breadmaking process reached its apogee in Britain in 1961 with the invention of the Chorleywood method of factory breadmaking, which could produce bread quickly, cheaply, and in stupendous quantities. The resulting white sliced loaf is made from flour that has had most of its nutritional value removed, and a combination of numerous additives added, including enzymes and a vastly increased proportion of yeast, which speeds up the breadmaking process and increases the shelf life of the bread. It is still the most common method of producing bread industrially in Britain today and, with some variations, around the globe.

So, the scales have turned almost completely and now it is white bread that is the cheap staple for the masses while whole-grain, and slowly produced, more nutritious breads, tend to be more expensive and are less readily available. Appearances can be deceptive, though, as many supermarket loaves that appear to be healthier are still highly processed. While they offer more nutritional value than a processed white loaf, they do not compare with the nutritional or digestive advantages of traditionally made bread because of the additives used and the rapid speed of production.

If factory-produced bread were to disappear overnight, there is no way that existing local bakers could meet the demand. For example, in the UK, around 80 percent of the bread that is bought is mass-produced, sliced, and wrapped. In-store bakeries in supermarkets account for 13 percent and the remaining 7 percent is bought from small bakeries.

Low-cost, processed bread is also one of the most wasted foodstuffs: it is estimated that one in every three slices of bread ends up in the trash. But if we are to move away from the status quo, one of the ways that we can start to change the economics and culture of breadmaking is to look differently at bread itself. Can we stop thinking of it as a disposable, cheap commodity and start to think of it as something that can be precious and nutritious? Can we move toward a new age of valuing bread as the staff of life? Yes we can—if we start to bake it ourselves.

> Can we stop thinking of bread as a disposable, cheap commodity and start to think of it as something that can be precious and nutritious?

DON'T YOU TELL ME WHAT TO EAT!

I don't like being preached to and I don't know anyone who does. The unhealthy eating habits that prevail across much of the planet exist despite the wide availability of good-quality information about what our bodies need, particularly from public sources such as health services. Their only vested interest is in reducing illness and consequent health expenditure. Why do we ignore the information that could save our lives? As well as the natural tendency to reject bossy advice, there are at least two other factors that cloud our judgement about what to eat and what to give others to eat.

The first one of these is the unrelenting pressure we are exposed to from commerce, food manufacturers, and retailers that want us to buy their products. The second influence is our emotional relationship with food which, as with most of our adult tendencies, will have its roots in our childhood experiences. What I have found to be useful in making better-quality decisions about what I eat is to understand better the way this emotional aspect of eating behavior works. This then makes it easier for me to work out what is going on, remember what works, what a good diet actually is, and look after myself better. I hope this can be helpful for you too.

THE GOOD NEWS

This chapter on nurturing yourself by eating well could have been extremely short. Something along the lines of the food and health writer Michael Pollan's belief that we should: "Eat food, mostly plants, not too much." On the other hand, it could have been a lengthy, scientific litany of dos and don'ts about what we should or should not be eating and why. It's okay—that won't be happening. The good news, and the reality, is that the most verifiable dietary advice is already familiar to us, and it is relatively straightforward.

Choosing to bake your own, high-quality loaves is an important step you can take to improve your diet and your health.

A balanced, healthy diet is composed of vegetables; whole grains; legumes; nuts and seeds; a modest amount of other proteins in the form of meat, fish, eggs; and dairy products; and some good fat (such as olive oil) and fruit.

There is no disputing that our health is also supported by reducing our intake of refined carbohydrates, trans fats, sugar, and salt. One of the easiest ways of reducing our intake of these problematic ingredients is to limit our intake of processed foods, most of which contain some or all of them. Manufactured bread is a processed food made from refined flour and many additives. Choosing to bake your own high-quality loaves is an important step you can take to improve your diet and your health. Just as importantly, turning your back on factory-made bread is a positive statement of commitment to improving your self-care.

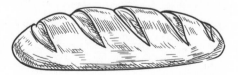

FALSE NEWS

Despite the basic message about what we need to eat being clear, it is often hidden behind competing communications from purveyors of processed foods or the proponents of fad diets. We are inundated with simplistic, sometimes contradictory, often misleading messages about what we should be eating. A very good instance of the truth being lost in an oversimplification lies in the way carbohydrates, as a food group, have been portrayed as bad for us.

Bread is often included in a broad condemnation of carbohydrates, yet the important distinction between "good" and "bad" carbohydrates sadly gets forgotten. Just as there are good fats (such as those found in nuts or oily fish) and less good fats (such as the trans fats found in processed products), so there are good and bad carbohydrates. The difference between good bread and bad bread is colossal.

We are subjected to a constant barrage of marketing from food manufacturers that use words like "farm," "country," "fresh," "natural," and "pure" to suggest to us that their products are nutritious and healthy, yet this is often far from the truth. Mass manufacturing processes lead to many foodstuffs being stripped of their nutritional value.

Poor nutrition is one of the factors implicated in the increase in chronic illnesses seen in countries where these processed foods are widely consumed, listed by the World Health Organization as obesity, diabetes, cardiovascular disease, cancer, osteoporosis, and dental disease. This nutritional deficit has led to a new and surprising phenomenon: obesity accompanied by malnutrition.

People are being seduced by food manufacturers and low prices, encouraged to fill up with empty calories from food made from refined flour and fat with salt and sugar or artificial sweeteners, and they are missing out on the essential nutrients only found in real food. So, to hear the quiet, clear lesson about what is good for us to eat, we need to start to be able to filter out the cacophony of multiple phony sales messages.

OUR COMPLEX RELATIONSHIP WITH FOOD

Our relationship with the food choices we make is also a function of our emotional state and our "food history." By food history I mean the way we have related to food and the messages we have been given about food in the past; both influence our eating habits. Some of these habits are a product of our individual experiences and some are culturally driven. Think about our tendency to use sugar-laden foods as rewards or treats. The associations we learn from being told: "be good and you can have some sweets," or "eat your vegetables or you won't get any dessert," can later lead to a habit of cheering ourselves up with a cake. Sugary foods then feature in our minds as something desirable and, paradoxically, as a way of nurturing ourselves. The sugary seduction we experience is played to in advertising that uses the "naughty but nice" message to encourage us to indulge ourselves.

The false news of old habits and advertising means that we might feel that we are being kind to ourselves if we eat a large bar of milk chocolate or a couple of doughnuts. Sometimes this leads to a repeating pattern of comfort eating, leading to self-criticism,

One of the most important ways we can both nurture and care for ourselves is by choosing to eat food that does us good in every sense.

which leads to more comfort eating and round and round it goes. The short-term gain of the sensory pleasure from eating sweet/salty/fatty/refined foods is followed by a long-term hit on our health and well-being. It is worth thinking about what being kind to ourselves really means when it comes to our food choices. If we really want to treat ourselves well, then we need to recognize that we deserve the best-quality food we can lay our hands on. By doing this, we are sending ourselves the hackneyed but true message that we are worth it. Eating real bread is a way of doing this and nurturing ourselves.

REDUCING EMOTIONAL EATING

Nurture is defined as caring for and protecting something or someone while they are growing.

Self-care is the practice of taking an active role in protecting one's own well-being and happiness, in particular during periods of stress. One of the most important ways we can both nurture and care for ourselves is by choosing to eat food that does us good in every sense.

For all of us, our decision-making is driven by both the emotional and the more logical, rational parts of our brains. We need both. We function best if we have a good balance between our emotional and rational thinking. This is very true when it comes to our food choices. I am not talking about choosing to eat the occasional sugary cake or portion of chips, but a persistent tendency to eat too much sweet/salty/fatty/refined food to the exclusion of real foods. I am also not addressing issues of seriously disordered eating here. Although some of the same principles apply, it is very important that anyone who has seriously disordered eating seeks professional medical help.

If we know what we should be eating and we can afford to buy fresh foods, then it's likely that unhealthy eating is being determined by emotional thinking. It is this dominance of emotional decision-making that explains the addictive consumption of foods we know are not good for us.

If we really want to treat ourselves well, then we need to recognize that we deserve the best-quality food we can lay our hands on. By doing this, we are sending ourselves the hackneyed but true message that we are worth it. Eating real bread is a way of doing this and nurturing ourselves.

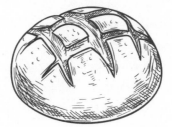

We can tell that this is what is going on if we find ourselves eating:

🌾 to reward ourselves for success

🌾 to console ourselves for perceived failure

🌾 to suppress negative feelings

🌾 to soothe ourselves at stressful times

🌾 to create a feeling of fullness or wholeness

🌾 as a response to boredom

🌾 as a comfort

🌾 to make ourselves feel better

🌾 to feel in control

It is worth noting that the same principle applies to the opposite: an obsession with healthy eating. This is another example of eating ceasing to be a way of looking after ourselves, a pleasure and a means to an end, but serving another emotional function. Orthorexia is an unhealthy obsession with eating healthy, pure, or "clean" food that is driven by a desire to manage negative thoughts and feelings and give a feeling of control.

I think it is helpful to think of the range of eating styles as being on a continuum. At one end is a poor-quality diet driven by emotional need, and at the other extreme is an unhealthy obsession with healthy food also driven by emotional need. As with so many aspects of human behavior, we are aiming for a happy medium, somewhere in the middle. What is helpful is to balance our emotional thinking about food with rational thought. The most powerful way of doing this, if we want to improve our

Do you think some of your eating behavior is emotionally driven in an unhelpful way?

🌿 Try keeping a food diary so you can identify any patterns.

🌿 Get into the habit of regularly checking in with yourself and naming your emotional state.

🌿 Get into the habit of asking yourself if you are eating something for an emotional reason.

🌿 Be clear about the emotional needs you are using food to meet and develop alternative, adaptive ways of providing yourself with what you need. For example, if you are eating for comfort, try a hot bath, reading, meditation, or talking to friends instead.

diets and eating behavior, is to try to separate our eating decisions from our emotional state. This doesn't mean we shouldn't enjoy food; quite the opposite: Mindfully eating nourishing food is deeply pleasurable. It does mean that our decisions about what and when we eat should be governed by being hungry, by what our body actually needs, by our own preferences, and by understanding what constitutes good nutrition. We then can enjoy our food and eating for its own sake rather than as an ill-fated strategy to manage our mood or anxiety level. As we move away from emotional eating, we then need to identify other ways of managing our emotional well-being that are adaptive, that don't cause us harm. Everyone is different, but we all have positive things we can do to ground and soothe ourselves. Opposite is a list of suggestions for you to start thinking about what might work for you, to help you ground and self-soothe.

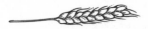

There is a wonderful win-win that arises when we bake our own bread. As well as providing a healthy contribution to our nutrition, the process of making bread allows us to slow down; it can be one of the ways we can manage anxiety and mood. Breadmaking gives us a sense of achievement as well as a concentrated loaf of nutritional goodness.

WHY IS REAL BREAD SO GOOD FOR ME?

By now you will be clear that all bread is not equal. Overly processed, factory-produced bread is not very good for you and there is evidence that consumption of refined carbohydrates has a negative health impact. At the same time we are understanding more than we ever have before that unrefined carbohydrates, in the form of whole grains, are actively good for our health. It is also the case that, in addition to its delicious and complex taste, bread made with a sourdough starter and allowed to ferment for an extended period of time has real advantages in terms of its digestibility. Let's have a look at the physical health benefits of real bread.

To start with, if you make your own bread, you will be spared the numerous additives, including enzymes, which are used in

Grounding, relaxing, and self-soothing activities

🌿 *Meditating*

🌿 *Walking in nature*

🌿 *Going for a run*

🌿 *Listening to music*

🌿 *Writing in a journal*

🌿 *Reading a novel*

🌿 *Talking to a friend*

🌿 *Relaxation and breathing exercises*

🌿 *Watching a movie*

🌿 *Going to the gym*

🌿 *A long, hot bath*

🌿 *Craft or arts activities*

🌿 *Gardening*

🌿 *Cooking, including baking bread*

Make a list of things or activities that have helped you in the past to manage your mood or anxiety level.

_____

_____

_____

manufactured bread to increase its softness and shelf life. For example, reading from the label of a processed loaf made with seeds, as well as the flour, yeast, seeds, salt, and added vitamins, the loaf also contains distilled vinegar, emulsifiers (mono- and diacetyl tartaric acid esters of mono- and diglycerides of fatty acids, mono- and diglycerides of fatty acids), preservative (calcium propionate), palm oil, and flour treatment agent ascorbic acid. Making your own bread means that you know exactly what is in it and it will not include these additives.

For a long time we have known about the importance of fiber or "roughage" for our health. It used to be thought that the fiber was inert and exerted its benefits simply by providing bulk, easing the passage of our gut contents through our digestive systems. We now also appreciate the more complex way in which fiber interacts with our gut microbiome—the mass of bacteria that occupies a healthy digestive system and supports our immune system, our mental health, and many other aspects of our physiology.

One of the most significant aspects of the impact of bread on our health is through this relationship with our microbiome. Wheat bran and oats are both very effective prebiotics, that is, they provide sustenance for the healthy bacteria we want to encourage in our guts. This can be enhanced even more by the addition of seeds, such as flaxseed, to your bread mix.

Refined white flour is the light color it is because the bran and the wheat germ have been removed from the whole grain. Using whole-wheat flour means that the bran and the wheat germ are still there and you will get the nutritional benefit of all parts of the grain. Ideally, choosing stone-ground as opposed to machine-milled flour will maximize this benefit. This is because flour that is ground traditionally with stone is not exposed to the high temperatures that are generated by the metal rollers in larger mills. The heat can damage some of the enzymes in the flour. Factory-made white bread has some nutritional additives put back into it, but it is impossible for the manufacturers to replicate the number and complexity of the micronutrients present in whole-grain flour. As well as being a very good source of dietary fiber, whole-grain bread provides us with a number of B vitamins and iron, manganese, zinc, and magnesium.

As well as the sort of flour we use, the nutritional value of the bread we eat is also influenced by the chosen method of proofing, which is what causes the bread to rise and expand before baking. The different methods of proofing all create bubbles of gas inside the pliable, raw dough, and when the bread is baked, steam is produced inside the dough, which continues the rise.

One of the things that is special about sourdough bread is that it has only three ingredients—flour, salt, and water. Sourdough gets its name from the pleasantly sour taste that comes from a lengthy, natural fermentation. Fermentation is the process in baking by which yeast and bacteria convert the sugars and starches found in flour into carbon dioxide. Instead of baker's yeast being added to the dough, a sourdough starter (see page 94) is used to ferment the dough over a much longer time. The activity of the sourdough starter—the creation of bubbles of gas in the dough—comes from the naturally occurring wild yeasts and lactobacilli in the flour, the air, the water, and the skin of the baker. The added ingredient to the flour, salt, and water in sourdough is time. It is this protracted fermentation or proofing time that has a major effect on how we digest the bread. The lengthy fermentation process helps to break down and change elements of the flour to a more digestible form, so for many people who struggle to digest mass- and fast-produced bread, sourdough can be better tolerated.

Time also plays a part in the role real bread can have in helping us to manage our weight. The complex carbohydrates in bread made from unrefined flour take longer to process and keep us feeling full for longer after we have eaten it.

A VIRTUOUS CIRCLE

So, eating real bread can reap rewards for us physically as part of a healthy diet. It can also aid our mental health, because looking after ourselves well, including eating a good diet, helps to establish a virtuous circle where we treat ourselves with compassion and respect. Looking after ourselves accordingly feeds positively into our self-esteem. Eating well is good self-care; good self-care is part of self-compassion; self-compassion aids good self-esteem, which in turn contributes to good mental health.

We know that becoming obsessed with healthy eating can become a real problem for some people. If we apply perfectionist tendencies to any area of our lives, then the same sorts of difficulties can arise. Instead of being something that enhances our lives, the obsession with healthy eating, for example, becomes a source of anxiety. One of the best ways of keeping our interest in healthy eating or healthy living in proportion is to remember that it is not an end in itself. Keeping well, being well-nourished, is something that enables us to have the energy, the strength, and the vitality to live the sort of life we want to live. Keeping well and eating healthily is the means to this end, but if it becomes an end in itself then we are missing the point. It would be like spending all our time polishing and oiling and tuning a bicycle and never going out for a ride on it. Like the ducks and the swans on the lake, the reason for eating a varied, natural diet is not to feel pleased with ourselves. Eating well enables the birds and us alike to have the means to live the full lives we are meant to live.

The following recipe is for a loaf of whole-grain bread that is super-charged with goodness. While tasting delicious, it will also keep you satisfied for hours, feed your gut biome, and provide you with many important phytonutrients.

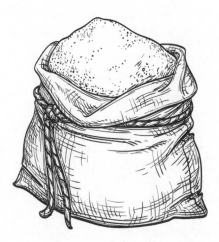

Whole-grain emmer seeded bread

Many of the ancient grains our ancestors used were nutritionally superior to strains of wheat grown today. You might need to do a bit of research or shopping around to find some of these more unusual flours, but it will be well worth the effort. This recipe is for a loaf made of nutrient-rich emmer flour, further fortified with seeds that add texture and even more nutritional punch. There are many ancient varieties of grain and flour that can be found at mill shops, delicatessens, health food stores, and specialty baking suppliers. As well as emmer, they include einkorn, spelt, teff, millet, farro, and khorasan. If you can't obtain emmer, then whole-grain spelt flour will work well.

Seeds are very concentrated sources of nutrients; this loaf contains pumpkin, sunflower, and nigella seeds, which provide extra fiber, trace elements, and protein.

This loaf will keep well for three or four days. If you think you might not need to use it all, you could freeze half for another time.

Makes 1 large loaf in a 9 x 5½-inch (1½ lb) pan, or 2 small loaves in 8½ x 4½-inch (1 lb) pans

INGREDIENTS

4¼ cups (18 oz/500 g) whole-grain emmer flour, plus extra for
   the pan(s) and for dusting
1 envelope (2¼ tsp/7 g) fast-acting yeast
1 tsp sugar (any type)
½ tsp fine salt (unrefined sea salt if possible)
1 tbsp pumpkin seeds
1 tbsp sunflower seeds
1 tsp nigella seeds (black onion seeds)
1½ cups (350 ml) warm water
1 tbsp oil (I use cold-pressed canola or olive oil—organic
   ideally), plus extra for greasing

METHOD

1. Stir together the flour, yeast, sugar, salt, and seeds in
   a large mixing bowl.

2. Mix the warm water and oil in a measuring cup.

3. Using a tablespoon, mix the water and oil into the dry
   ingredients in the bowl until it starts to come together
   into a rough ball.

4. Begin the kneading in the bowl until the dough is
   holding together, then continue to knead on a lightly
   floured work surface for 5 minutes (you can take rests

if you need to, nothing bad will happen). You might find you need a little more flour as you go, but try not to add too much.

5. Put the dough back into the bowl and cover the bowl with a damp dish towel, making sure that the cloth doesn't touch the dough. You can fasten the cloth with clothespins.

6. Leave the dough to rise for 1 hour.

7. Prepare your pan or pans by greasing the inside surfaces with a small amount of oil using a paper towel. Then dust the pan(s) with flour to cover these surfaces.

8. The next stage is called "knocking back." It means working the dough to remove some of the gas produced in the first rise and will enable flavor and an even structure in the bread's "crumb" (see page 56) to develop. You can do this by pressing the dough out into a flat shape.

9. Now it is time to shape the dough. Fold the dough in on itself and then roll it and shape it to the approximate size of your pan(s) and gently put the dough into the pan(s) with any seams or joins underneath.

10. Leave the dough to rise in the pan(s) for another hour, again covering it with a damp cloth to avoid a dry skin forming on the surface.

11. Heat the oven to 400°F/200°C.

12. Bake for approximately 40 minutes in the center of the oven, by which time it should be golden brown and be producing the lovely smell of baked bread.

13. Using oven gloves to hold the pan, tap the base of it sharply on a worktop to help loosen the bread. If the loaf seems to have come loose, gently tip it out on to a dry dish towel and knock the bottom of the loaf with your knuckle; it will sound hollow if it is done. If you feel it needs a little longer in the oven or you want to brown the sides more, put it directly on to the oven shelf for another 5 minutes. If you have any difficulty removing the loaf from the pan, then you might need to, very gently, run a thin knife between the loaf and the pan.

14. Allow the bread to cool on a cooling rack before slicing and eating.

Reflect on how you have used unadulterated and natural ingredients, heat, time, and your own hands and energy to make a nutritious loaf of bread that would be recognized by your ancestors millennia ago: real bread that is really nutritious and nourishing.

There are so many ways you can eat your bread: toasted, with jam or in a sandwich, but sometimes the simplest things are the best. One of the most satisfying and enjoyable things we can do with our homemade bread is to remind ourselves of the perfect pairing—a slice of bread and butter.

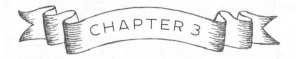

CHAPTER 3

Being Creative

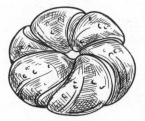

Just as a musician learns the rules of music before attempting improvisation, once you are reasonably confident about the basics of breadmaking then you will be ready to start experimenting and trying variations. Getting stuck in our ways and staying with what we know is something we all tend toward. Doing the same old thing does have some merits, not least familiarity, confidence, and comfort. But we pay a price for staying within our comfort zone and being on automatic pilot. We limit our potential for growth and change and we can miss out on the benefits of creativity. To make things creatively is life-affirming, mood-enhancing, and satisfying. The feeling of flourishing we can achieve when we pull a beautiful

To make things creatively is life-affirming, mood-enhancing and satisfying.

loaf of bread out of the oven can stay with us for some time and spread into other areas of our lives. Experimenting with our breadmaking can make it easier for us to take a chance on other things too. Creative activity can foster a sense of achievement and well-being and it does not have to be artistic or problem-solving to count as creative. Making your own bread falls squarely into the category of everyday creativity—positive activities that can be used by anyone to improve their well-being. There is a wonderful, virtuous circle possible here in that the better you feel, the more likely you are to make the effort to make things, to be creative; and the more you exercise your creativity, the more positive your mood and sense of self-worth—and, in addition, you have something beautiful and nourishing to show for it.

CREATIVITY AND A GOOD SENSE OF SELF

As well as making us feel better, being creative feeds a strong and positive sense of self. By creating something that is personal, we are putting something out into the world that reflects who we are. When we make something, we can see ourselves mirrored in the thing we have created outside of ourselves. When we then see how the object we have made, whether it be a loaf of bread, a painting, or a piece of craftwork, is received and appreciated by others, we recognize other people's enjoyment of our creation and this reflects back to us, supporting our sense of who we are. This deep benefit of being creative is powerful because it echoes the fundamental process in infancy by which we develop our sense of self in the first place. It is by attunement with our emotional state, and then mirroring this back to us, that our mother or primary caregiver enables us to develop both a sense of ourselves and of the validity of our emotions. By being soothed, we also learn how to self-soothe. Picture a crying infant and an attuned mom instinctively making a sad face back to the child as she acknowledges (long before the child is verbal): "Oh, poor you, you're upset, there-there, let's have a cuddle." By repeating back to an infant their facial expression or the tone of what they have said, the parent can convey to the child that they have been heard and that their emotional state has been understood. If, for whatever reason, we have not had good enough parenting in this respect, then creativity is one of the ways we can make up for it and effectively re-parent ourselves. By creating something and offering it to others, we are echoing the child's offering of words and emotion to their parent; in taking in others' responses to our creation we are providing ourselves with validation. By creating bread from flour, water, and salt we are able to both literally feed ourselves, and others, and metaphorically feed our healthy sense of self, our identity.

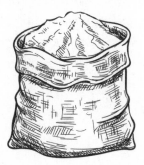

CREATIVITY, CURIOSITY, EXPERIMENTATION, AND INVENTION

Making bread by hand can be a way of expressing ourselves creatively. We start with recipes that allow us to develop our understanding of the baking processes, but once we have mastered these fundamentals then we are free to think about options and choices, and there are so many.

Composing combinations of ingredients is what this is all about. Get daring: start to develop your understanding of the different flours and flavors and how you might combine them. Sometimes experiments will work incredibly well, other times you may not want to repeat them. A sculptor or artist needs to develop an intimate knowledge of their materials and their qualities and idiosyncrasies. They need to know how different materials combine or react to changes in the environment. The artist learns about materials by trying things out. This is how you will find out about your ingredients and breadmaking processes too.

I have an old cookery book from the 1960s that is tall and thin and has its pages sliced horizontally into three sections. The idea is that you pick a first course from the top, a main course from the middle and a dessert from the bottom. You can flick the separate sections of the pages to mix up what goes with what. I could imagine a similar arrangement for experimenting with bread. The three sections to be shuffled and experimented with in bread-baking are:

- raising method
- flour
- additions, such as herbs or seeds

The possibilities that follow are for savory breads. There is another whole range of possibilities in enriched or sweetened doughs (in which fat, eggs, or sugar are added) that are not covered here. These breads include brioche or croissants. I think for now, there is more than enough scope for us to exercise our creative muscles with basic doughs, but you might want to experiment with the richer and sweeter doughs another time, as your skills develop.

The descriptions in the following list of possible bread ingredients will help you to think about novel combinations you might like to try, as well as tried-and-tested combinations, such as cheese and onion or potato and dill. Just like an artist, as a breadmaker your knowledge about the differing characteristics of the many elements at your disposal will grow. You will also start to get a better sense of which ingredients go well together, both in relation to taste and the effectiveness of the proofing and baking processes. Creative experimentation is the best way to grow your expertise in what works and what creates the best-tasting breads for you and the people you bake for.

RAISING METHODS

"Leavened bread" is the term that covers all breads that include a raising agent. A raising agent is what allows the dough to expand during proofing. Unleavened breads are flatbreads, such as naan bread, or crackers, like matzos, that are made only from flour, salt, and water (and are not left to ferment like sourdough). Unleavened bread does not rise.

There are three main methods for producing leavened bread and they all involve the production of gas (carbon dioxide). The gas produced forms bubbles in the gluten structure of the dough, which stops your loaves from being solid bricks. These bubbles can vary from enormous cavities, such as in white sourdough, to modest, little bubbles in whole-grain bread. Both are fine and reflect the varying gluten content, water content (this is called hydration), and density of the flours. This texture and the distribution and size of holes inside a loaf of bread is called the "crumb." The three methods of raising bread range from soda bread, which rises instantaneously, to yeasted bread, which takes a few hours, to sourdough, which takes at least a day or more.

Baking soda is the basis for a rapid method of raising bread dough. The best-known version of this is Irish soda bread. Instead of being produced by either baker's or naturally occurring yeasts, the carbon dioxide, which creates the open crumb of the loaf, is produced by the chemical reaction between the baking soda and the acid in the dough in the form of buttermilk, yogurt, or milk mixed with lemon juice. It really is instant, so much so that it is important to get the loaf into the oven as soon as it is mixed. Using this method of raising, you can produce a freshly baked loaf of bread from scratch in under an hour.

Yeast is a microorganism, and it would be more accurate to refer to "yeasts," as there are many varieties of them more or less everywhere. Yeasts are present in the air and on many surfaces, including human skin. Whenever you see fermentation, you will know that yeasts are present. Yeast will make your dough rise as long as it is provided with three essentials: food—in the form of simple sugars (derived from the flour), warmth, and water.

There are three main forms of yeast available to the baker: fresh (or "cake") yeast, dry yeast (sometimes called "traditional" or "active dry" yeast), and a more concentrated, powdered form of yeast that is variously called "fast-acting," "bread machine," or "instant" yeast. Both dried and instant yeasts can be stored for long periods of time. Baking yeasted breads involves one or usually two proofing periods where the dough is kept in a warm place for some hours to allow the yeast to ferment to produce the gas which will aerate your bread.

Fresh yeast, also called "cake" yeast, will stay usable for up to two weeks in the fridge, but will lose its power if it gets much older. It has the appearance of slightly crumbly putty. Fresh yeast is 100 percent pure but, for many of us, lack of availability and short shelf life make using it a rarity. It is used by crumbling it into warm water with some sugar or honey until it starts to bubble.

Dry yeast (it is sometimes called "traditional" or "active dry"), has the appearance of tiny pellets or granules. Again, it is 100 percent yeast and it needs to be dissolved in warm water before it can be used. This "proofing" process (allowing the yeast to start to ferment) takes about 15 minutes. The warm water activates the yeast and it should start forming a froth on the water it is mixed with.

Instant yeast (which is sometimes labeled "fast-acting" or "bread machine") is a powder that you just add straight to your dry ingredients. Unlike fresh or dried yeasts, instant yeast contains additives. It is more concentrated than dried yeast, which is in turn more concentrated than fresh yeast.

You will discover that bread recipes will refer to yeast or baker's yeast in any of these forms. They are all interchangeable, so don't worry if you have a different sort to the one mentioned in an ingredients list as long as you convert to the right quantity and use the correct mixing method.

A rule of thumb for converting amounts of yeast is that for 4¼ cups (18 oz/500 g) of flour, you would use either 1 cake (.6 oz) of fresh yeast, 1¾ tsp (5 g) of active dry yeast, or 1 tsp (3 g) of instant (fast-acting) yeast, though recipes do vary.

Sourdough bread is also made with yeast, but it is made with wild yeast that naturally occurs on the flour. The naturally occurring yeasts and lactobacilli (helpful lactic acid bacteria) that multiply in the dough are responsible for the fermentation, which results in carbon dioxide being produced, which in turn lifts the dough. The sourdough process takes at least 24 hours. Bakers often choose to leave their sourdough developing for a longer time in a cool place to improve flavor. It is this lengthy fermentation that leads to the characteristic sour taste. Once the sourdough process is established, it is self-perpetuating, as a portion of the starter is kept back to begin the dough-making process the next time. Whichever flour you use to make your sourdough starter, you can use the same or a different sort of flour to mix your main dough.

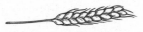

FLOUR

Looking at the array of flours available can be a bit overwhelming. There's all-purpose flour, self-rising, bread flour, organic, stone-ground, whole-wheat, white unbleached, white, brown, multi-grain, malted—it is a long list. Let's start with the two variables that apply to flour produced from any variety of grain. If you want to maximize both the purity and the nutritional content of the bread you make, choosing to use flour that is both organic and stone-ground is a great first step.

Organic flour is produced from grain that has been grown without pesticides or herbicides and will not have been made from genetically modified crops. Whichever sort of flour you are buying, seeking out an organic version will ensure that the flour is free of these sorts of contaminants.

Stone-ground flour is produced in smaller quantities than its machine-milled counterparts and is therefore more expensive. I would argue that the higher price is worth paying for both the superior taste and nutritional value of this sort of flour. Industrial milling methods involve metal rollers revolving at high speeds. The bran and the germ—the parts of the grain that contain much of its nutritional value—are removed early in the process. The heat produced by the speed of the rollers then further denatures some of the remaining nutrients in the resulting white flour. Because of this, millers are obliged by law to add nutrients, such as vitamins, back into their flour. Stone-ground flour has a number of advantages over the machine-milled version. Grinding the grain with stones produces much less heat so the nutrients are not damaged. The process produces whole-grain flour and if the traditional miller wants to produce white flour, then this is sifted at the end of the procedure. Because the endosperm (the starchy center of the grain) is milled along with the bran and germ, some of the nutrients are absorbed by the endosperm during the milling. If the miller is making whole-grain flour, then you can be sure 100 percent of the grain is present. If the industrial miller is making, for example, whole wheat flour, they have to add back the bran and germ which were extracted at the beginning of the industrial process and there is no guarantee it is actually whole-grain. Whether you choose to use whole-grain or white flour (or a mixture of both), then using stone-ground is best for both taste and nutritional value.

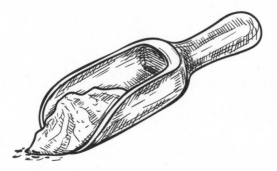

CHOOSING YOUR GRAIN

Now that you have decided on the type of flour you will be using, you also need to think about the sort of grain the flour has been made from.

Wheat is the most commonly used grain for producing flour and it comes in many varieties and strains. Varieties of wheat vary in their protein content. Protein content is important as it influences the amount of gluten produced in the dough made from the flour. The gluten is important in allowing the dough to rise, producing a good crumb in the bread. Types of wheat that have a high protein content are described as "hard" and the flour produced from them is called bread flour. It is possible to make good bread from flour that is lower in protein like all-purpose or a mixture, but when starting out, if you are making bread from wheat flour, then looking for bread flour is helpful. Bread flour will rise well. Weaker flour from softer wheat (like cake flour) is perfect for baking cakes and pastry.

Whole-wheat flour contains the bran, which does not contribute to gluten production, so this flour tends to rise less than all-purpose or bread flour. Bread made from 100 percent whole-grain wheat will taste lovely and will be quite dense. Many bakers will use a mix of whole-wheat and bread flours to balance the nutritional value and taste with the rising qualities of the white flour. This will produce a good-tasting loaf with a more open crumb texture than all whole-wheat. One of the many variables you can experiment with is the ratio of whole-wheat to white flours in your bread mix.

Rye is grown across the north of Europe and is often used to bake traditional, sourdough breads; it is a nutritious grain with a high soluble fiber content. It ferments quickly, which is one of the reasons it is also used in making whiskey. Rye flour does contain some gluten but not as much as wheat flour. Again, a loaf made from 100 percent whole-grain rye would be quite heavy and dense (which some people love). For a lighter loaf, a mix of rye with another flour higher in gluten works well. Pumpernickel bread is made from rye flour and rye meal (a more coarsely ground grain). Experiment with the relative proportions of rye and white bread flour until you get your own favorite ratio.

Spelt is an ancient grain and is actually a species of wheat. It is often the most readily obtainable ancient grain. Spelt has a high fiber content and often a higher protein content than other wheats. Bread made from this grain tends to rise more quickly than bread made of flour from conventional wheat. But because it has less glutenin (a form of gluten) than other wheat flours, it needs less working and kneading than other doughs. Spelt is often considered easier to digest than other wheat flours, but it does still contain gluten. Spelt flour produces a creamy, mild-flavored bread and works very well in the sourdough process.

Einkorn, emmer, and khorasan are also in the wheat family and are ancient grains. Khorasan (sold under the trade name Kamut), like spelt, has a high protein content with less efficient gluten formation and, also like spelt, seems to be more easily digested by people who are sensitive to contemporary wheats. It is perplexing that proponents of a "Paleo" diet advocate avoiding grains, as einkorn is very similar to grains eaten by our ancestors at that time. There is archaeological evidence that at the end of the Palaeolithic period, wild grains were being harvested. Both einkorn and emmer produce a good-flavored bread that doesn't rise quite as much as bread made from modern flours, but is no worse for that. Other ancient grains include teff, sorghum, and freekeh.

Oats and barley are both highly nutritious grains with cholesterol-reducing qualities. Although not completely gluten free, they are not hard enough flours to add any volume to a bake and for this reason are best used as part of a mixed-grain recipe. What they do add is excellent flavor and a softness of texture.

Gluten-free flours are not a new thing and are available in numerous forms. They can be made from nuts; legumes, such as chickpeas, corn, rice, coconut, and buckwheat (not related to wheat); or even green bananas. There is an extremely good argument for baking your own bread and other baked goods if you need to follow a gluten-free diet. This is because most manufacturers of gluten-free baked products pack them with additives used to try to replicate the tastes and textures of equivalent products made with gluten. Ready-made, gluten-free baked products may be bought for health reasons, but actually can be highly processed and full of artificial ingredients, so not quite as healthy as might first appear. If you decide to bake your own gluten-free bread, you will know exactly what is in it. It is obvious, but worth pointing out, that gluten-free bread will not be the same as bread that has gluten in it. Regard this as an opportunity to be really creative. Instead of seeing gluten-free bread as a pale imitation of normal bread, see it as a chance to experiment with good-quality ingredients to create something different and new. The lack of gluten does mean that the texture of the bread will not be chewy or stretchy; it will be more cake-like, but a gluten-free loaf can still taste brilliant.

The process is going to be different too. The reason we knead dough is to develop the gluten, so no gluten means no need to knead. The dough you make with gluten-free flours will need to be fairly wet and in some cases can more or less be poured into your lined baking pans. Often the most successful gluten-free loaves are made from a mixture of gluten-free flours to make the most of their differing tastes and textures.

Managing our expectations in baking and life leads to calm acceptance. Calm acceptance is a great way of avoiding anxiety. Your gluten-free bread will be different from bread that contains gluten and it will be good.

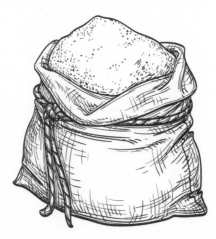

ADDITIONS

This is where we come to the potential for almost limitless per-mutations. In thinking about the possible additions to your savory dough, it is worth thinking about what you want to achieve. Do you want to enhance or change the flavor of the bread? Do you want to change its texture or color? Do you want to increase the nutritional content of the bread? If you are adding a vegetable, moisture is a consideration and can be an issue. Adding a vegetable can be a great way of keeping the crumb soft for longer, but too much wetness, for example from grated zucchini, can lead to soggy bread. Hard vegetables such as potatoes, squash, or carrots work well grated raw into the dough.

The lists below are a starting point for you to explore, experiment, and be creative.

Through trying out new combinations, and depending on where you are in the world and your personal preferences, you will be able to develop your own list of ingredients to add to your bread. Keep a record as you go so you can note which recipes and ingredients work best for you.

Seeds

Adding seeds is one way to improve both the taste and nutritional value of your bread. The seeds will add weight to the dough and may inhibit its rising if you add too many, so the proportion of seeds is something for you to experiment with. Adding up to a quarter of the weight of seeds to flour works well for most seeds, for example a mixture of flaxseed, sunflower, and pumpkin seeds. Some seeds such as caraway have a very strong taste and a small sprinkle is enough.

Nigella (black onion) seeds impart an incredible, savory taste to bread and, again, you don't need too many of them—a teaspoonful for a large loaf would be ideal.

The following seeds deliver on taste, texture, and nutrition. You can add one of them, all of them, or any combination in between. I often make a whole-grain sourdough loaf with a mix of the first eight of these seeds and it tastes wonderful.

- sunflower seeds
- pumpkin seeds
- sesame seeds (golden and black)
- nigella seeds
- flaxseed
- poppy seeds
- golden linseed
- fennel seeds
- cardamom seeds
- caraway seeds
- cumin seeds

Nuts

Adding nuts to your dough can also add taste, texture, and nutrients to the bread you are making. It is best to chop or crush the nuts before incorporating them into the dough. Try:

- walnuts
- almonds
- pecans
- cashews

Bran

Adding bran is an easy way of increasing the fiber content of your loaves, something that is very good for the health of your gut. Bran is the outer covering of grains or seeds and, as well as providing soluble fiber, it is rich in nutrients, including fatty acids and B vitamins. Try:

- oat bran
- wheat bran
- rice bran
- corn bran

Herbs

Adding herbs is a wonderful way to add flavor to your bread. Chopped, fresh herbs are ideal, but dried ones work well too. For some herbs, mostly those with a softer leaf, you will find that you will need to use a larger quantity than you think as the baking process can mute their taste. Hardy herbs, such as rosemary and thyme, retain their strong flavor even when cooked. Think about the food you will be eating the bread with and use herbs that pair well with it. Bread made with dill, for example, is great with fish, while chives complement cheese. This is yet another area in which to exercise your creativity. Try:

- basil
- chives
- dill
- rosemary
- sage
- thyme
- oregano

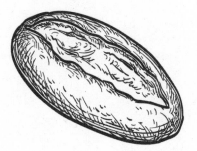

Oil or butter

Adding oil or butter to your bread dough will influence the crumb (the inner texture of the bread) as well as the taste. Oil "shortens" the gluten strands, making for softer bread that also stays soft for longer. We are just talking about a quick glug of oil here, not too much. If you want to add oil to your dough, then it is probably worth thinking primarily about the impact on the taste of your bread. The following oils will add taste as well as having a crumb-softening effect.

- olive oil
- walnut oil
- pumpkin seed oil
- sesame oil

Spice

Adding spices to your dough can transform your bread in subtle ways. You can also go the whole hog and use spices, if you are so inclined, to make your loaves taste like curry or pizza—you name it, you can bake it. Choose the spices you would normally add to a dish and experiment away! Turmeric or paprika will alter the color too.

- ginger
- fenugreek
- nutmeg
- chili powder
- turmeric
- cardamom
- cumin
- coriander
- paprika

Cheese

Adding cheese produces a lovely, savory bread. Freshly grated hard cheese can be added to the flour at the beginning of the process. Use roughly 4 oz of cheese for 3½ cups of flour. Cheese with onion or chives works very well with soda bread or a yeasted loaf. Try:

- Cheddar
- Parmesan
- hard, smoked cheese
- Manchego
- pecorino

Vegetables

Adding vegetables to bread dough might sound a bit odd, but it is a great way to use up old root vegetables that may be lurking in the bottom of the fridge. It is also a good way to improve the taste, texture, and keeping qualities of the bread produced. As ever, when adding ingredients to dough, it is important to be mindful of both the additional water content of the ingredients and the impact on gluten formation. Adding grated raw root vegetables is a good way to start experimenting with vegetables in bread. The water content is relatively low and keeping the vegetable to flour ratio to approximately three parts grated vegetable to five parts flour works well. When using softer vegetables, such as tomatoes, it is better if the tomatoes are dried or semi dried. Onions, garlic, mushrooms, or peppers that you intend to add to dough are best fried first, both for flavor and to reduce their water content. Try:

- potato
- beet
- carrot
- onion
- celeriac
- garlic

- olives
- squash
- tomatoes
- sweet potato

- pumpkin
- spinach
- mushrooms

Of course, not everything will go with everything, but there is huge scope for creativity and experimentation in trying out combinations from the lists above.

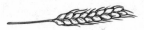

The two recipes that follow will give you a good start with two vegetable breads that incorporate either soft leaves (basil or wild garlic both work well in place of the spinach) or grated root vegetables. Once you have tried these recipes, you will be able to let your imagination take you to new variations and combinations. There is one flatbread—a green spinach tortilla—and a yeasted bread made with grated raw beet that is tasty and looks amazing with its purple spots.

Spinach Flatbread

There are only four ingredients in this unleavened bread that makes healthy wraps. You will need a mixing bowl, a small pan, a blender, and a heavy-bottomed frying pan or cast-iron skillet. If you have a stick blender, then use this with a measuring cup, otherwise use a regular blender. The mixture starts off being bright green, but becomes less lurid when cooked.

Makes 12

INGREDIENTS

2 cups (8½ oz/240 g) whole-grain spelt flour, plus extra for
   dusting
½ tsp fine salt (unrefined sea salt if possible)
3½ oz (100 g) baby spinach
¼ cup (60 ml) water

METHOD

1. Mix the flour and salt in a large bowl.

2. Place the spinach in a pan with the water over medium heat and cook until wilted.

3. Transfer the spinach and its water to a blender. You should end up with about 1 cup (230 ml) of liquidized spinach; add a little more water to make up the volume if necessary.

4. Mix the blended spinach with the dry ingredients and knead gently into a ball of dough.

5. Form the dough into a log shape and divide into 12.

6. Dust your work surface with a little flour. Roll each piece of dough into a ball, then dust it with a little more flour, before rolling out into a thin disc, about 6 inches across. The dough can be a little sticky, so you can use a dough scraper or spatula to lift it.

7. Heat a large, heavy frying pan and dry fry each tortilla for 1–2 minutes on each side. As they cook they will turn darker green and brown spots will appear.

8. Wrap in a cloth or foil to keep warm and to stop them drying out before eating. Like other flatbreads, these are best cooked and eaten fresh, but the wrapped dough will keep in the fridge for a day or so.

Dill and beet bread

(adapted from Dan Lepard's recipe for Dill and Potato Bread, first published in the *Guardian*)

There is something particularly pleasing about the earthy taste of beet, the buttery smell of baked dill, and the glorious colors of this bread. Slicing into it is a revelation. It provides a feast for the senses and will give you a well-deserved sense of achievement. When I first baked Dan Lepard's Dill and Potato Bread, from which this loaf was inspired, I knew it was a recipe I would treasure and use for the rest of my life. You might think that raw potato or beet would make for soggy bread, but not at all. This is a loaf that is full of flavor and whose crumb will stay soft for days.

You will need a mixing bowl, a coarse grater, and a baking sheet with baking parchment to make this recipe. It will take around 20 minutes to prepare and mix the dough, then this will need to rest for 90 minutes. After shaping, the loaf will then need another hour of rising before being baked for 45 minutes, so about 3 hours and 35 minutes in total.

Makes 1 loaf

INGREDIENTS

½ envelope (1 tsp/3 g) fast-acting yeast
a large bunch of dill, finely chopped (you can substitute dried
    dill if necessary, use a good tablespoon full if you do)
1¼ cups (275 ml) warm water
12 oz (350 g) peeled, raw beet, grated
5 cups (21¼ oz/550 g) all-purpose flour, plus extra for dusting
2½ tsp salt (unrefined sea salt if possible)
3½ tbsp (50 ml) olive oil

METHOD

1. In a large mixing bowl, stir the yeast and chopped dill
   into the warm water.

2. Add the grated beet, then stir in the flour, salt, and olive
   oil. Mix well, then leave to stand for a few minutes.

3. Work the dough in the bowl with your hands for a few
   seconds—it won't feel like a normal dough, but don't
   worry. You are aiming to get it to come together in a ball
   rather than actually kneading it.

4. Cover with a damp dish towel (this stops the dough
   from drying out and forming a skin, which would
   interfere with its rising) and leave for 90 minutes at
   room temperature.

5. Turn the dough out on to a floured work surface and shape it into a ball.

6. Line a baking sheet with baking parchment and place the dough on it with the seamed side underneath.

7. Cover with the damp dish towel and leave for another hour.

8. Heat the oven to 425°F/220°C. Gently rub some flour over the surface of the risen dough (rubbing it rather than just dusting it helps it to stick) and score a line or cross into the surface, then place in the oven for 45 minutes.

9. Let the loaf cool completely on a cooling rack before cutting into it. You will be tempted because the smell is wonderful.

Now you can start improvising. Be daring; invent something new; take chances—you can always experiment with reduced quantities. Fill your kitchen with the warm smells of herbs and seeds and spices. Create nourishing and delicious loaves from combinations of ingredients you've never tried before. Surprise yourself with what you can create with your own hands and imagination. Use the process of making bread to free your mind.

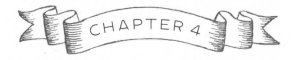

CHAPTER 4

Lifelong Learning

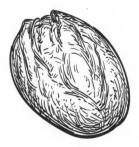

Learning to make bread is a journey that never ends. It is telling a story that never finishes: this is wonderful. It means that you can never know everything there is to know about the art and science of baking bread, so you can keep on learning about it for as long as you live. In the process of this perpetual learning, unlike the ancient alchemists who failed to turn base metals into gold, you will learn many ways of turning flour and yeasts and water and salt into golden globes of deliciousness. No matter how many recipes and techniques you learn, there will always be more to learn. Believe me, this is such a good thing. Learning about making bread can be a project that accompanies you through the rest of your life.

Starting to learn something new can give us helpful insights into ourselves and our attitudes to learning. This can give us a chance to address any fears or insecurities that belong in our past. We can also learn to bake bread as a meditation, as an exercise in mindfulness and devotion. By becoming engrossed in the task of baking, we are engaged in an activity that involves continually developing skills and learning. This is a recipe for being in a state of "flow"—in "the zone," or completely focused and energized by a task or activity. Being in this state is one way we can achieve a real sense of satisfaction with our lives. Continuing to learn is also one of the ways we can help to maintain our cognitive capacity as we grow older. Concentrating on learning about one area or set of skills, such as breadmaking, can provide us with a lifetime of focus and stimulation. Sometimes, the narrower the field we focus on, the more intensely we become captivated by the details and potential for further learning.

LEARNING TO KEEP AN EYE ON YOURSELF: A BASIC AND ESSENTIAL SELF-HELP TOOL

If we are facing a task or challenge, then it is really helpful if we can be mindful of how we are thinking about it. This might sound odd, but we are not our thoughts or, indeed, our emotions. There is a part of us that can observe what we are thinking and feeling. Getting better at being an accurate observer of our own mental, physical, and emotional states is one of the most useful skills we can develop on the road to knowing ourselves and growing into being the best version of ourselves we can manage. Meditation and mindfulness are our allies in this.

Being able to notice, identify, accept, and then—if we so desire—change what we are thinking, provides us with the potential to manage and regulate our emotional states and influence our actions. Socrates told us that an unexamined life was not worth living. Developing the skills of being able to examine ourselves and our lives can be transformative.

Being fully aware of our own thinking and feelings gives us tremendous freedom to shape and influence our own lives. The converse—living an unexamined life—means that we are more or less on automatic pilot. We are at the mercy of habitual thinking patterns and emotional responses which will have been developed in our formative years and which may well be serving us ill now.

By learning to notice and acknowledge what we are thinking and feeling, we buy ourselves the freedom to choose. We can either choose to keep on thinking, feeling, or doing the same old thing or we can choose to think, feel, or do something differently. We can choose to think, feel, or act in more adaptive ways, in ways that are more balanced and that demonstrate self-compassion. This is not necessarily an easy process but, like making sourdough bread, it is absolutely worth the effort.

Whenever we want to create psychological change in ourselves, the starting point is knowing where we are now. It is only when we tell ourselves the truth about where we are now that we can begin to adjust and make changes. It is never too late to start to learn how to be a better observer of ourselves and it is therefore never too late to begin to make changes. We can stop being our own worst enemy and start treating ourselves as we would treat a friend or a vulnerable child: with kindness.

It is never too late to start to learn how to be a better observer of ourselves and it is therefore never too late to begin to make changes.

So how can we learn this skill? How can we learn to be a better observer of ourselves? How can we pave the way for psychological change and growth?

You have everything you need to start this learning process right now. You are going to be able to switch on a new level of awareness that will afford you new freedoms and the potential for further change.

Your observer is already there; they have been there all along. The exercise opposite will help you wake them up and encourage their attentiveness.

"WHAT IS GOING ON HERE?"

Once we have become used to checking in with our bodies, thoughts, and emotions regularly, we can start to ask ourselves whether these thoughts or feelings are appropriate. A very straight-forward definition of good mental well-being is to be feeling the appropriate emotion at the appropriate time in the appropriate intensity. This means that there are times when feeling sad or angry is a perfectly fitting response to the situation we are in. When our response is appropriate, then it is important that it is not repressed; we need to think and feel and process what is going on for us. This allows us to act accordingly and move on. But if we recognize that the response is not appropriate; if, for example, the idea of making

Reflective exercise—becoming your own observer

As often as you can remember to do so, check in with yourself by answering the following questions—they will wake your inner observer and encourage them to be alert.

🌿 *What am I feeling in my body right now? Am I feeling tense, fidgety, hungry, thirsty, relaxed, agitated, tired? Recognize what you are physically feeling, name it, and acknowledge it to yourself.*

🌿 *What thoughts have just gone through my head? What am I saying to myself? Am I worrying about something? Am I dwelling on something from the past? Am I concerned about something in the future? Am I criticizing myself? Recognize what you are thinking, name the sort of thinking, and acknowledge it to yourself.*

🌿 *How would I describe my emotional state right now? Am I scared, angry, happy, contented, sad? Recognize what you are feeling emotionally, name it, and acknowledge it to yourself.*

This is a practice that needs to be learned. If we learn it well, it will become second nature to us and we will have created a new, healthy habit of mind. Many of us have ignored our inner observer for so long that they have fallen asleep. We need to learn how to rouse them and get them working for us.

sourdough bread leads us to feel scared, thinking, "I won't be able to do this, I'll make a mess of it, I haven't got the patience, I'll look like a fool," then there are further questions we can ask ourselves about the way we are thinking. We can ask ourselves:

🌿 *Is this helpful?*

🌿 *Is thinking or feeling like this what I want or need right now?*

🌿 *Is thinking or feeling like this taking me nearer or farther away from being the person I want to be and doing what I want to be doing in my life today?*

As well as the regular checking in with yourself, it is also helpful to use any occasions when you start to feel upset in any way as a prompt to consult your observer. The universally useful questions to ask yourself/your observer are:

🌿 *What is going on here?*

🌿 *What am I reacting to?*

🌿 *Does this response belong in the here and now?*

🌿 *Is there another way of thinking about this?*

🌿 *What would I say to a friend in this situation?*

In other words, we all have a choice about how we think about, feel about, and react to things. It has taken me a long time to learn these lessons too. My habitual response to any sort of disapproval or criticism used to be to feel crushed and worthless. But slowly, by recognizing what I was thinking (*I am stupid*), how I was feeling (*hopelessness*) and reacting (*giving up*), I have been able to find a way to face these things in a much less defensive and personal way.

In approaching a new skill, such as making bread, our attitude will be influenced by our earlier experiences of learning. For many of us, our experiences at school will have been mixed. If we have grown up believing that discovery is fun, making mistakes is normal, and that we can learn just about anything if we put our minds to it, then it is likely that we will face a new experience with excitement and optimism. If, however, we have learned that we mustn't make mistakes and should be able to master something right away, that if something goes wrong people will judge us, or if we do not succeed, then it is because we are not good enough, then we will naturally countenance this new task with trepidation and pessimism.

If you find yourself contemplating making sourdough or any other bread with anxiety, then ask yourself what thoughts are going through your head. Challenge those thoughts. They don't belong in the here and now. Remind yourself that no one is going to judge you. You can do this. The worst that can happen is that your bread might be soggy or split or stuck to the pan, but it will still be edible. The best that could happen is that it all turns out well right away. The most likely is that you will have hitches and ups and downs, but will get there in the end. Anxiety is fed by avoidance, so the best way to counter anxiety is to face the thing you are afraid of and get baking!

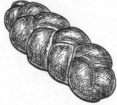

LEARNING ABOUT YOURSELF: BAKING YOUR WAY TO A JOYFUL MIND

In devoting time and energy to developing your practical knowledge about breadmaking, you are also going to have the opportunity to make discoveries about yourself. If we think about the monastic life and the devotional approach to mundane tasks, such as cleaning, or we consider how we often get good ideas when we are out on a long walk, we realize that some of our most helpful and profound psychological and spiritual learning comes when we are engaged in sometimes repetitive, physical tasks. I think this is particularly true for activities that take us closer to nature. These are the activities that allow us to sink back into the universal, to have a sense of our connection with the earth, with people who have gone before us and those who will follow. Iris Murdoch, the philosopher and novelist, talked about a process she called "unselfing," a stepping outside the self with a humble and non-judgemental attitude. At the simplest level it means losing ourselves in nature or art—being taken out of ourselves. It has much in common with mindfulness.

> Some of our most helpful and profound psychological and spiritual learning comes when we are engaged in sometimes repetitive, physical tasks.

We can learn to make our bread-baking a meditation. In that absorption, attention to detail, and care for what we are doing, we can learn to let go of our worries and of ourselves. In this way, by giving breadmaking our full attention, we can master a helpful way of managing our stress levels and start to learn to access an inner peace.

There is much to learn in this respect from the attitude to food preparation in Buddhist communities. In a monastery, the *tenzo* is the monk who is given responsibility for feeding the whole group. If we look at the role, it becomes clear that this is much more than a mundane job. The tenzo is required to put their whole self to work and to the tasks required of them with a joyful and awakened mind. The tenzo is required to handle all of the ingredients needed for the day's meals with great precision, care, and respect. No matter how senior or enlightened the monk, the tenzo must roll their sleeves up and wash the rice and prepare the vegetables themself, paying full attention to their task. Likewise, however humble the food being prepared, the same respect and reverence for the ingredients and process must be adhered to. Making a thin vegetable soup is as worthy of full attention and care as a more elaborate or rich meal. The joyful mind comes from throwing all passion for life into the work of cooking. The spirit in which the tenzo's work is done transforms the activity. Some texts even encourage the cook to treat the food as a parent cares for their child.

How could you apply this approach to your breadmaking? Could you choose and handle your equipment and ingredients with tenderness and care? What would it feel like to direct your full attention to the task at hand? Could you learn to give your whole self to the process of making your bread? Could you think of your ingredients and bread as being precious like a child? Could you make bread-baking your route to a joyful mind?

It is not necessary to have any particular spiritual beliefs to be able to adopt this focused attitude to breadmaking and to benefit from developing a joyful mind yourself.

LEARNING TO FIND FLOW IN BREADMAKING

There is another way of looking at the learning process of bread-making that also helps us to see how it can be something that contributes to living a calm, enjoyable, and fulfilled life.

Fascinated by artists who got lost in their work, the psychologist Mihaly Csikszentmihalyi came up with the concept of "flow" to describe a state of mind and being, which he identifies as being a stepping stone to a sense of fulfillment and even happiness. Have you ever been so engrossed in an activity that you lost track of time? That you forgot about yourself? The chances are that you were in a state of flow.

According to this way of looking at flow, one of the conditions which makes it more likely to be experienced is being in a learning situation, where there is a reasonable balance between our skills and the requirements of the task, but where we are still being stretched. For example, I might be a painter who is confident in her painting skills but who has never tackled a particular subject before. I think learning to make bread can readily provide us with this sort of circumstance. Learning to make bread can be part of a virtuous circle where the learning process leads us to experience a sense of flow, which in turn feeds into our personal development and growth, which then contributes to our happiness and our desire to learn and bake more bread.

Like our artist who has a clear idea of what she is aiming for in her painting, having a goal for what you want to achieve is another beneficial condition for achieving flow. But we also need to have a realistic view of what the challenges might be. If you have the goal of becoming a regular baker of sourdough bread, then you will need to face certain necessary tasks, such as learning how to cultivate a sourdough starter, how to feed it and keep it alive, baking techniques, and starting to understand the nature of different doughs. This means developing skills. To develop skills you need to be able to monitor your progress and start to recognize the impact of the exercise of these skills and other factors on the taste, rise, and texture of your loaves. To do this, you need feedback and, for many bakers, keeping a record of their different bakes is the way to do this. You can record the weight of ingredients (and if you want, the relative proportions), rising time and temperature, baking time and temperature, and then a description of how the resulting loaf turned out. This is a brilliant way of learning from your accumulating experience.

In learning to bake bread, you can be reminded again of the joyful mind of the tenzo and of Iris Murdoch's "unselfing." In giving your full attention to the task of learning how to make bread, you can achieve flow, mindfulness, and a healthy losing of yourself. Achieving this sort of single focus is something that you can continuously improve. Keeping your awareness on what you are doing requires regular realigning of your attention. Distractions present themselves either from the outside world or from your own thoughts, and the challenge is to notice this and pull your attention back to what you are doing.

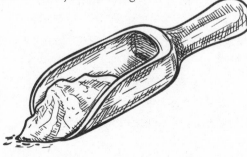

TRAINING OUR ATTENTION

Being able to better control our attention gives us the freedom to wrest it back from thoughts and scenarios over which it is not in our best interests to ruminate. In giving our attention to the task and the learning, we lose self-consciousness and we can enter a state of flow.

Understanding flow takes us back around to mindfulness and another level of satisfaction and peace with our lives. This ability to redirect, to train where we put our attention, is—like developing our inner observer—another fundamental building block of good emotional health. There is a sense in which our reality, our consciousness, is formed of what we choose to give our attention to. One of the reasons depression and anxiety are so debilitating is that they rob us of our attention and drag our focus into worrying thoughts and past or predicted catastrophes. But when we learn to set goals, to develop skills and learn from feedback, to learn how to direct our attention and immerse ourselves in what we are doing, we have the potential to find joy in everything and anything. This does not, of course, mean that we will be protected from loss, disappointment, or hurt, but that we are less likely to be defeated by the inevitable suffering that is an existential reality for all of us. Also, if we put effort into identifying goals and a sense of purpose in our lives, then flow can become the way we live our whole life. Whatever we are doing, the activity can be enhanced by being in the moment and by giving it our full attention. Like an artist who is completely engaged as they sculpt or paint, we can also cultivate the ability to be more absorbed and focused on what we are doing, whether we are cleaning or cooking or cycling or swimming or walking.

Then if we have identified a sense of purpose, it can impart another layer of meaning to these everyday actions. Our artist might have a determination to honor and create beauty as her reason for getting up in the morning. By letting this inform her everyday life as well as her artistic work, she is able to generate a sense of cohesion and harmony, whether she is at her easel or washing the floor. When I mindfully make bread for my family I am expressing my purpose of letting them know they are loved. Learning to be in the moment and learning to recognize what we really care about can lead us to one of the most precious gifts we can give ourselves: the knowledge that we can transform our experience by training our attention and understanding our sense of purpose.

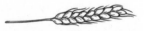

LEARNING A CRAFT

The Japanese word *shokunin* means "craftsman" or "artisan." There is a renowned sushi chef called Jiro Ono who has had a celebrated documentary film made about his life's work in which this notion is explored. It is a universal quality of a craftsperson's approach that the devotion goes beyond the mastering of technical skills. The shokunin makes a commitment to perpetual improvement and refining of their craft, and to work tirelessly for the honor of the craft itself as well as the people who will benefit from it. In the film, *Jiro Dreams of Sushi*, the elderly man talks about the need to immerse yourself in what you are doing, making an effort and repeating the same thing every day—the need to fall in love with your work. We can fall in love with making bread, and although we may not be able to devote ourselves so completely to the process, we can, like Jiro, approach it as a mountain to be climbed, whose top we know we will never reach. This may sound slightly dispiriting, but it doesn't need to be. Whether we are making sushi, painting pictures, or baking bread, no matter how skilled we become, there will always be more for us to learn. In accepting this, we can choose to devote ourselves to continuous development as we learn our craft.

Could you embark on an unhurried commitment to getting better and better at making bread? To make it with love and dedication for people that matter to you? To know that the perfect loaf does not really exist, but that one can spend a lifetime getting closer to it?

Craftsmanship involves the desire to do things well and a dedication to learning. It can fulfill our need to keep ourselves connected to material reality. The craftsmen involved in building great buildings, such as cathedrals, spent their whole working lives dedicated to doing the best job they possibly could, and there is something about craftsmen's pride in their work which is inspiring to me. One story about craftsmanship sent tingles up my spine when I first heard it. Stonemasons who worked on the restoration of a great cathedral uncovered a workmen's room, high up in a hidden roof space of the vast church. This was a place where tools were kept—a place that no one but the workmen would ever see, yet they had made beautiful carvings there. They had made something that was an expression of their craft, not for human praise, but for its own sake. There is something profoundly moving to me in this idea that we can do our best, be dedicated to doing something really well for the sake of the craft itself, rather than for praise or reward.

Learning how to make good bread is something that we can dedicate ourselves to for its own sake, as well as it being a means to many beneficial ends. The rest of this chapter is dedicated to setting you on the path to becoming a craftsperson of sourdough baking.

LEARNING TO MAKE SOURDOUGH BREAD

It is completely normal when you first start to learn a new skill or delve into a new area of knowledge to feel out of your depth. Making sourdough bread is a skill that has sometimes been given the reputation of being difficult and unduly time-consuming and therefore, maybe more than other types of baking, people shy away from it. It is true that it takes longer than making yeasted bread, but the flavor and satisfaction that come from transforming flour, water, and salt into sourdough bread is absolutely worth the time and effort. The instructions that follow will guide you through the process step by step.

Expect to feel unsure and unconfident at first, know that you will make mistakes and that some attempts will not turn out as expected, and remember that this is fine. It is all part of the learning process and the more you make sourdough, the more your confidence will grow. It is also important to remember that even for the most seasoned bakers, there can be mishaps and miscalculations; it is normal.

The difference with sourdough

The big difference between making sourdough bread and making bread with yeast is that the first stage of sourdough baking requires the making of a "starter," sometimes also referred to as a "culture," "mother," or "chef." Flour and water are mixed together and encouraged—with warmth and time—to ferment. Naturally occurring yeasts and bacteria on the flour will transform the white paste into a living broth, which is kept in a plastic container or ceramic or glass jar with a loose-fitting lid. As fermentation involves the mixture expanding, the container needs to have enough room for this to happen, and too tight a lid on a fragile container could result in it shattering. Whenever you make sourdough bread, you will use a portion of this starter to mix with flour, water, and salt to create an active dough that will rise well.

Making a starter can take up to a week, but often it will be ready to use after four days, and you only need to make it once, as the sourdough baking process involves saving some of the starter each time you bake, ready to feed and keep it for the next time.

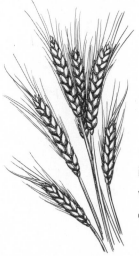

Potentially your starter will live for years! Some people claim to have starters that have been bubbling away for decades.

It is quite difficult to kill the starter once it is going. It is normal for your starter to become dormant; it enters this state when you put it in the fridge, for example, but refreshing it— by feeding it—will wake it up. It may look as if it is dead, with no bubbles and a gray/brown, watery liquid on top, but it is unlikely to be dead. Mixing it up, feeding it, and placing it in a warm place will almost always do the trick and wake it. Most bakers wouldn't leave their starter unfed for more than two weeks. If you want to leave it for longer, your starter can be frozen.

Excessive heat (using water that is too hot, for example) is one of the few things that can kill your starter, but this is easily avoided by testing the temperature of the water before it is added—aim for no warmer than 95°F (35°C). One other problem can be contamination with unwanted molds or other organisms from the air or utensils, although this is rare because the acidity of the starter produced by the healthy bacteria and yeasts usually inhibits the growth of less welcome microorganisms. You will know that this has happened if you notice a different, unpleasant smell or if there is pink, green, or dark brown discoloration on your starter. If the worst happens and your starter goes bad or dies, it is not a disaster because you can just throw it out and make another one.

So the first stage of making sourdough bread is making your starter, and this is something that, once done, will only need to be repeated very occasionally, if at all. The remaining stages of sourdough making will be repeated every time you bake and in between to ensure good maintenance of your starter. I will suggest a routine for incorporating sourdough baking into your busy life, but ultimately you will find out what works for you; we are all different. The instructions that follow are gleaned from a number of sources including my own trial and error and a beautifully straightforward method taught to me by food writer Orlando Murrin. This method is a simple one. No one owns the recipe for sourdough bread; it has been made by our ancestors for millennia. At the back of this book are suggestions for further reading about sourdough baking where you will find variations on the method (see page 176).

There are a number of additional possible stages to making sourdough loaves, which you may want to graduate to in the future. Reading these books, written by expert bakers, is another of the ways that you can go on learning and developing your own skills and style of sourdough baking. For now, though, this is the easiest sourdough loaf possible. There are two parts to the following directions on making sourdough bread. First there is a section on what you will need and how to make your starter. Then there is a section on what you will need and the recipe to use some of your starter to make a loaf of sourdough bread.

HOW TO MAKE A SOURDOUGH STARTER

It is possible to buy commercial, dried sourdough starter or you can be given some of someone else's starter to use. While there is nothing wrong with these ways of getting your hands on a starter, I think there is a great advantage to making your own. There is something very personal about having your own starter and, at the beginning of what could be a lifetime of using it, working with your own from the very start of your sourdough journey is important because you are deeply connected to something you have made yourself. While this may sound a bit "out there," trust me, it's true.

This is what you will need:

A suitable container
This can be a wide-necked glass jar, a plastic tub with a lid, or a ceramic pot with a lid. You can use a cloth or plastic cover for your pot if you prefer. It is important to cover your growing starter to

keep unwanted organisms out, but also to avoid sealing it too tightly so that gas doesn't build up in the container. Metal containers are best avoided because of possible chemical reactions. Using a transparent container does have the advantage of letting you see the slow developing activity of your starter. Thoroughly wash and rinse your container before you start.

Water

If you are lucky enough to have water that isn't from the mains, then you have a head start. If you are using chlorinated tap water, leaving a pitcher of it to stand overnight will allow most of the chlorine to evaporate away before you use it. Water that is of medium hardness is best for bread-baking. While it's not always easy to gauge this, if you know that your tap water is either very hard or very soft, then using bottled still spring water would be best. When you are making and refreshing your starter, use warm water (up to about 95°F/35°C).

Flour

The visible ingredients that make up your sourdough starter are flour and water. What makes a starter active are the invisible ingredients—the wild yeasts and lactic acid bacteria that come from the grain the flour was milled from. The wild yeasts produce gas (carbon dioxide), which helps the dough to rise, and alcohol, which evaporates during baking; the bacteria produce lactic acid which adds to the flavor and stops any unwelcome organisms from growing in the starter. Organic, stone-ground flour from grain that has not been treated with chemicals and that has been ground without excessive heat will be richest in these yeasts and lactic acid bacteria, so it is worth using either whole-grain wheat or rye flour to make it—both are great. Rye ferments very well and you don't have to make rye bread from it; the flour you use to bake will determine the sort of sourdough you produce.

Heat

Keeping your growing starter warm enough is important at this stage (it will be able to cope well with cold once it is up and running). The ideal temperature is 75 to 85°F/25 to 30°C. This is warmer than the room temperature in most houses, depending on where you live in the world. Possible good spots are in a closet near a hot water tank or near a radiator or a stove. You can also wrap your pot of starter in a blanket to conserve warmth. If the temperature is a bit cooler than the ideal, then there will be no harm done, the fermentation will just take longer, as long as it is warm enough to get started. Avoid direct heat, the yeasts you want to thrive can't survive at temperatures above about 140°F/60°C and you don't want to kill them off.

Time

Depending on the other variables such as warmth, a starter will take as long as it takes until it is ready to be used to bake with— anything from four days to two weeks. Once you have mixed your flour and water, you are going to feed it every 24 hours for as long as required.

A sourdough starter

METHOD

1. Pour 1 cup (4¼ oz/120 g) flour (see page 95) and 1 cup (250 ml) warm water into your clean container and combine using a wooden spoon.

2. Put the container, covered but not sealed, into a warm place for 24 hours.

3. Now you are going to feed your starter, and you will need to keep feeding it every 24 hours until it is ready. Before you feed your starter, throw half of it away. You can do this by eye—there's no need to weigh it. (Once you get past the starter-making stage, you can find other uses for what is called the "discard," such as making crumpets or crackers.) Add ½ cup (125 ml) warm water and ½ cup (2⅛ oz/60 g) flour to the remainder in your container and mix with a wooden spoon. Return to the warm place for another 24 hours.

4. Repeat this feeding process until you notice evidence of fermentation. It will start to expand and creep up the container; there will be bubbles and you may notice a pleasant beery or sour smell. When you can see a bubbly froth, your starter is done. It might take only 4 days to reach this stage or it can take up to 2 weeks, at which point you should have a pale, slightly bubbly starter with a consistency like a thick batter.

WHAT YOU WILL NEED TO MAKE YOUR SOURDOUGH LOAF

- a banneton or proofing basket—the banneton is made of cane and the concentric rings create a lovely ridged pattern on the risen dough. You can also get purpose-made proofing baskets which are lined with linen or you can improvise one with a round basket and a cotton or linen napkin.

- a lame, razor blade, or sharp knife for scoring (see page 103)

- a medium bowl

- a large mixing bowl

- a measuring cup

- a dough scraper

- a large, cast-iron Dutch oven (optional)

A sourdough loaf

To make sure your starter is primed for baking, it is worth giving it a double feed.

The following timings lead up to your sourdough bread being baked approximately 24 hours after you have first mixed your dough. Your dough will sit for half the time at room temperature and then, when shaped, will spend the night in the fridge.

The double feed: if you have been feeding your starter in the evening, the day before you plan to mix your dough, give the starter an extra feed at lunchtime or in the morning. Remember these timings are a rough guide, you do what fits best with your own routine. For example, you might give your starter an extra feed during the day on Friday (or on Friday morning); feed it as normal on the Friday evening, then mix your dough first thing on Saturday morning, let it rise for 12 hours, then shape it and let it rise for a second time overnight in the fridge on Saturday. You will be ready to bake your loaf on Sunday morning.

Your choice of flour will determine the character of your sourdough bread. White bread flour will give you a lighter and airy loaf with holes in the crumb and a hard crust. Whole-grain flour will produce a denser loaf with a softer crust. You can mix any proportion of flours to achieve the sort of loaf you and your family like to eat.

Makes 1 loaf

INGREDIENTS

4⅓ cups (18⅓ oz/520 g) flour (I use a 50:50 mixture of
   whole-grain and unbleached all-purpose flours, see page 59),
   plus extra for dusting
¾ tsp fine salt (sea salt if possible; see also page 182)
1¼ cups (300 ml) warm water
⅓ cup (85 g) starter (see page 97)

METHOD

Mixing

1. Mix the flour and salt together in a medium bowl.

2. Pour the warm water into a large mixing bowl and add
   the starter. All being well, the starter should semi-float in
   the water. Whisk or stir them together gently.

3. Now stir the flour into the water, mixing it with a
   wooden spoon. You might not need quite all of the
   flour or you may need a tiny bit more. Flours differ in
   how absorbent they are. If in doubt, err on the side of
   stickiness rather than adding too much flour—you are
   aiming for it all to hold together. Leaving the dough in
   the bowl, knead it gently, pulling the dough together for
   a few minutes to form a rough ball.

The first rise

4. Cover the bowl—you can use a damp dish towel or a plastic cover. Leave the covered bowl at room temperature for about 12 hours. In that time, the dough should roughly double in size.

Shaping

5. When the first rise is completed, gently turn the dough out on to a lightly floured work surface and gently fold it in on itself and turn it around to form a taut ball of dough. The smooth surface will be uppermost and there will be seams and a bit more untidiness underneath, this is fine.

The second rise

6. For the next stage of rising it is best to use a banneton or proofing basket. Whether using a banneton or a basket with cloth you will need to flour the inside to prevent the dough from sticking. If you are using a banneton for the first time, the day before you use it, give it a spray with water and then a liberal dusting with flour (this is before the first use only). When you come to use the banneton, shake the excess flour off and give it a new, generous sprinkling of flour.

7. Carefully place the dough in the basket, smooth-side down. Cover and leave in the fridge overnight.

Baking

8. There are two options for baking your loaf. The first is to use a "Dutch oven." This is any large, cast-iron casserole with a close-fitting lid, which is heated inside the oven. The one I use is 12 inches across and 5½ inches deep. The second option, if you don't have a suitable cast-iron pot, is to bake the loaf on a baking sheet or baking stone. Both methods need a sheet of baking parchment with a sprinkling of flour. The advantage of using the pot is that, for the first half of baking, the steamy atmosphere produced allows the loaf to rise fully before, during the second half when the lid is removed, the crust is allowed to harden and color.

9. Heat the oven to 450°F/230°C. This might seem pretty hot, but bread ovens are usually hotter than this. If you are using a pot or stone, preheat this in the oven.

10. When the oven is just about up to temperature, put a sheet of baking parchment on your work surface (if you are using the pot or stone) or straight on to your baking sheet. Sprinkle the middle of the parchment with some flour over an area slightly wider than the size of the base of the loaf.

11. The dough in the basket should have risen a bit more. Very gently ease the dough away from the sides of the basket or banneton with your fingers before turning the loaf out on to the baking parchment. If it is at all stuck, again use your fingers to gently ease the dough away from the basket, holding it upside-down above the parchment.

12. It is not unusual for the dough to stick a little and it is not at all rare for the dough to start spreading at this stage, but try not to worry, getting it into the oven quickly is the best way of limiting this, but before this happens you need to score the surface of the dough.

Scoring

The reason for cutting lines into sourdough is not just to decorate it, although wonderful patterns can be made. Making a slash or slashes with a sharp knife, a blade, or a lame helps to control the way that a loaf expands and rises in the oven. The dough expands first during rising, then it expands again as it is being baked. This rise is called "oven spring" and it results from the steam that is produced inside the dough as it bakes. Without scoring, the loaf will split in an unpredictable, uneven way which can produce an oddly shaped loaf. The scoring controls how this happens and produces a more symmetrical loaf. A simple line across the center or a cross are a good way to start scoring.

13. Using a sharp implement, gently but firmly make a cut or cuts in the surface of the dough. It will start to open up immediately and this is fine.

Into the oven

14. If you are using a Dutch oven or baking stone, using oven gloves and with great care (it will be extremely hot) take the pot out of the oven, place it on the stovetop or a trivet and remove the lid. Pick the dough up with the ends of the baking parchment and lower it into the pot, replace the lid, and put it back into the oven. After about 25 minutes (halfway through the baking), using your oven gloves, carefully remove the lid from the pot. The crust will then brown and crisp in the final 25 minutes.

15. If you have put your dough straight onto parchment on a baking sheet, put this in the oven now. Ovens vary, but the loaf should be cooked in approximately 50 minutes.

16. You will be able to judge both the color and smell of a well-baked loaf as you get more used to baking sourdough. If you think the bread looks and smells done (and it has been in the oven for at least 50 minutes), then it is time to get it out. If using a pot, lift the pot out on to the stovetop and, using the baking parchment, lift the loaf out and slide it on to a cooling rack. Tap the base with your knuckle, if it sounds hollow, then this is another sign that the bread is done. The same applies if you have used a baking sheet.

Cooling

17. It might be tempting to dive into hot bread, but it is best to let it cool naturally, at room temperature, before tasting it. It will be easier to cut and will have better texture and flavor.

Congratulations. You have made a loaf of sourdough bread from scratch, starting with only flour, water, and salt and your time and care and attention. Well done. Enjoy it and feel a well-deserved sense of achievement. It may be that your loaf has turned out well or maybe it hasn't turned out quite how you expected, but accept it whatever its flaws—this is a learning curve. Celebrate your loaf in all its imperfect uniqueness.

SAVING SOME STARTER FOR YOUR NEXT LOAF

Keep the starter you have left over, give it a quick feed by discarding half of it and adding ½ cup (125 ml) warm water and ½ cup (60 g) flour, and then keep it covered in the fridge until your next baking day. If you don't bake very often, then feeding your starter once a week will keep it healthy.

TIMELINES

The more you make sourdough bread, the more you will develop your own routines and ways of fitting the different stages into your life. The following timelines will give you a good starting point and an easy reference.

Starter timeline

Day 1: make your starter.

Day 2: feed your starter by discarding half of it and adding more flour and water.

Days 3, 4, etc.: continue the feeding process every day until the starter is bubbly and increasing in size.

MAKING YOUR LOAF

1. The day before you want to make your dough, feed the starter in the morning and again in the evening.

2. First thing the next morning, mix and knead your dough.

3. Leave to rise in the mixing bowl for 12 hours. In the evening, fold the dough in on itself and gently shape into a ball.

4. Place it seam-side up in a proofing basket, cover with a damp cloth, and leave it in the fridge overnight.

5. The next morning, turn your dough out on to a floured sheet of baking parchment and score the surface.

6. Bake either in a Dutch oven or on a baking sheet or baking stone.

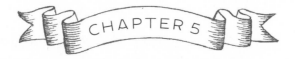

CHAPTER 5

Truth

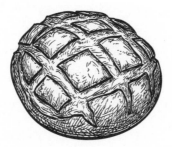

This chapter starts with bread and ends with bread. In the middle of this sandwich is an opportunity to think about what is important to us, what motivates us, and how an understanding of our values enables us to make choices that match up with what we really care about. I think you will now have a good idea why making and eating our own bread can make a positive contribution to our physical and emotional health and well-being as part of good self-care. Now I want to explore how making our own bread can also be an expression of our wider values in a way that, by adding to our feelings of integrity and fulfillment, can support our mental health and improve our quality of life.

THE VALUES IN A HOMEMADE LOAF

When I see the dark, nut-brown, lightly raised edges of the crust of a homemade loaf of sourdough bread, I can also see authenticity, kindness, beauty, quality, nurturing, nature, creativity, sustainability, care for the environment, slow food, patience, experiential learning, real food, hard work, dedication, perseverance, and simplicity. These are all things that matter very much to me and I see them all in the bread I make. The truth of my devotion to baking bread, in all its myriad forms, lies not only in the delicious taste and nutritional value, or even the process of making it, but also in what it stands for and represents to me. There is every chance that you will be able to see and express the things that matter to you too in making bread. This is because so many of the qualities and values of handmade bread, and the process of making it, are universal.

Everyday decision-making

From the moment we wake in the morning, we make decisions and choices. What will we use to wash ourselves? What will we wear? Will we listen to the news or not? What will we eat and drink for breakfast? How will we travel to wherever we are going that day? And how will we spend our day? The expression "spending time" is illuminating; it helps to give us a sense of time as something precious, a currency. This, in turn, makes it easier for us to value time and the importance of the decisions we make about how we use it.

How our values help us to make decisions

If we had to go back to first principles and examine all possible options every time we made a decision, then it would be so time-consuming—we would not be able to get through a day. In the absence of a rationale for decision-making, it could also be difficult to maintain a sense of self. There is a virtuous circle that comes about when we know who we are and what we believe in so that we then make decisions that agree with and reinforce this sense of self. Without this, it would be as if we remade ourselves anew every day with every decision. What we rely on are ways of rationalizing the way we make decisions. For example, if I am a vegetarian, I don't consider and reject the idea of eating meat at every meal. I have already made the decision and choose accordingly. We use a range of "operating principles" to simplify the decision-making process and to give meaning and consistency to our lives. The simplifiers include habit, ritual, beliefs, values, politics, religion, desires, memory, cultural norms, morality, rules, and assumptions. These principles allow us to feel there is some order to our decisions. What we do and how we live our lives is informed by them, so the choices we make all feed into our values and to our sense of self, our identity. Our vegetarian has made the decision that she will not eat animal products and this choice reflects her values. In turn these values and beliefs form part of the way she sees herself and her identity. Being a vegetarian is part of who she is as well, as what she believes in, and what she does. These three; how we behave, what we believe in, and how we see ourselves, influence and shape each other. It is rare to find anyone who has a perfect match between their identity, their beliefs, and their actions. Maybe people who have taken religious orders will most likely be able to achieve this sort of full integration. For the rest of us, there is a normal state of flux and muddle, contradiction and compromise. However, this is one of the aspects of our lives that we are free gradually to change.

Becoming more aware of our values is the route to improving the harmony between what we believe in, what we do, and who we are. This matters because moving toward more coherence between the everyday decisions we make, what we believe in, and our sense of self gives us a feeling of integrity and purpose.

THE LIMITS OF CHOICE

There are some things which we have no choice over. We all have aspects of our lives that are beyond our control. We have to eat, we have to drink, we have to sleep; we cannot choose the particular circumstances of our birth, our parentage, or where and when we are alive. We all die and we are all imperfect. We can't change these givens or these particularities, although we can choose to change how we see them or think about them.

We can also respond to these inevitable aspects of existence with some freedom. We have to eat, for example, but we can exercise choice about what we eat. We will all die, but some of us will be lucky enough to be able to make decisions about where and how we end our days. We have more freedom to choose than we sometimes give ourselves credit for. But, if we were genuinely open to all of our options at any one moment, we would be overwhelmed and probably immobilized by indecision—we would not make it out of bed in the morning! Our value systems therefore act as our guide to integrating what we believe in and the decisions we make.

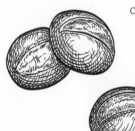

KNOWING OURSELVES

One of the many characteristics of people with good mental health is their ability to understand what really matters to them, what their values are and, then, as much as possible, to act in accordance with these values. From Socrates extolling the examined life, to our modern-day attempts—through therapy or contemplation—to understand ourselves better, there is a recognition that this matters. It is important to know what we stand for and what sort of a person we are. This might sound a bit odd, but we are not often called on to describe ourselves or explain what really matters to us. It is not always easy, but it is something that is helpful and that we can use to start to delve into ourselves.

We are not born with a ready-made set of beliefs and values. We learn them from other people, from our experiences, and from what we are taught by our families, our friends, our religious and academic teachers, and from society in our formative years. One of the characteristics of adolescence is the way we start to question and examine some of these beliefs. The rebelliousness of youth is a healthy sign that values and a sense of self are being negotiated. It is also a time when peers, social media, and ubiquitous advertising pile the pressure on young people to be a certain way, to fit in, to be accepted and included. Conflicting pressures can lead us to feel stress. These pressures do not stop when we reach adulthood, and the dynamic process of examining and re-examining what matters to us and what we believe in goes on too. It is important to know what we believe in because it gives us a yardstick against which we can assess the choices and decisions we make.

BEING AUTHENTIC

If we make decisions that agree with what we believe in, then we have a sense of authenticity, a feeling that we are being true to ourselves. The philosopher Søren Kierkegaard reminded us that: "The commonest form of despair is not being who you are." However fraught the odyssey might be to better self-knowledge, it is worth it because approaching it gives us a feeling of integrity and wholeness. The opposite, living our lives in a way that is at odds with who we really are, with what we believe in, is a cause of internal conflict, which can lead to anxiety, depression, and a feeling that life is pretty meaningless.

The most important thing to remember here is that we can go on improving our understanding of ourselves and our values throughout our lives. We are all familiar with people who transform their lives by making significant career changes. This is usually an indication that this person has understood something about themselves and their values, which has informed their decision. To change direction, to make these sorts of shifts, involves letting go of old values that are no longer relevant or important to the individual. It can be really helpful to ask ourselves if we are still carrying around values that we no longer believe in and maybe belong to someone else from our past. It may be that we have not really examined values that we have inherited from a parent, for example. We might have taken as a given that academic achievement and a professional career are necessary for a happy life, but it might be that actually what we really care about is being outdoors, working in nature or with our hands. This not recognizing that we are adhering to a family value we don't actually share, can lead to us feeling deep unhappiness and inner conflict as we try to live our lives according to someone else's rules.

Make a list and identify any beliefs you have been carrying around that you no longer believe in, that do not belong to you, and do not serve you now. Try identifying what you really think and believe in place of these

We can go on improving our understanding of ourselves and our values throughout our lives.

second-hand theories. Here are a couple of examples from my life to start you off. I was brought up to believe many things that I have since rejected and no longer recognize as having anything to do with my own values. A very pervasive idea was the belief that the worst possible thing I could do was to be selfish and that I should always put other people before myself. While I do value looking after others, being kind and compassionate, I also strongly believe that we should show ourselves the same kindness and compassion that we show to others. I think that unnecessary self-sacrifice and self-denial actually lead to resentment and unhappiness all around.

Another pernicious belief passed on to me was the certainty that whatever I did, it wouldn't be good enough. The message was clear: if I tried something new or that involved putting myself forward in some way, then the consequence would be the double ignominy of being seen to be both a show-off and a failure. Needless to say, it took a while for me to build the confidence and self-esteem to be able to move away from this belief, to risk failure and even risk success. I believe now that I am as capable as anyone else of good things and that we are all actually able to do much more than we realize.

Now you try; it is a good feeling to acknowledge that you have moved on.

UNDERSTANDING OUR DEEPER MOTIVATIONS

Beginning to understand what is going on beneath the surface is another valuable way of understanding ourselves better. It is important to remember that the sense of meaning in our lives is also a function of our unconscious needs and desires. By definition, these unconscious drives are hidden, but it is possible to deduce what they are. One of the ways you can start to think about your own unconscious motivations is to ask yourself:

What did I need when I was growing up that I did not get?

The likelihood is that you are still looking for whatever it was you lacked, or you are still mourning the absence of it now. It is also true that we will feel driven to give to other people whatever it is we were missing in our childhoods. The list of things we might have missed out on or didn't get enough of when we were growing up is a long one. It includes:

- love
- affection
- attention
- approval
- food
- stability
- structure
- boundaries

- a secure base
- fairness
- tranquility
- laughter
- freedom from violence and aggression
- being heard
- encouragement
- having our emotions acknowledged, understood, or contained
- admiration and praise
- kindness
- freedom to play
- freedom to make friends
- opportunities to learn

This is not an exhaustive list, but no matter how many words are on it, the impact of the deficiencies will be the same. We will be driven to keep searching for whatever it was we missed out on. We may also have our mood dragged down by the unexpressed grief we carry for the childhood we might have wished for but didn't have. Again, this striving is not a bad thing in itself, in fact it plays a part in the way we can recover and move on from the shortcomings of our upbringings.

But it is important to be aware of what is going on, so that we can understand and process and, if we can, accept the reality of what happened to us and what we missed out on. If we are not aware of how strong this urge is to find, for example, the affection we did not get sufficiently in childhood, then we may be prone to making poor-quality decisions about relationships, as our neediness clouds our judgement of who might be good for us as adults.

The awareness is also necessary to stop us repeating unhelpful patterns from our own childhoods. There is a risk that, without this awareness, we are on autopilot and unwittingly might repeat problematic ways we were treated by our parents or carers with our own children. Someone who had to adhere to strict rules and was excessively criticized as a child may find themselves imposing the same regime on their children, "for their own good." Of course, this does not mean someone is deliberately setting out to do something harmful to their children; it is more that, for someone with this experience themselves, being strict or harsh with children seems like a good idea, the "right" way to parent. Conversely, the fear of repeating their own experience can be so powerful that a parent might go so far in the opposite direction that other problems arise, for example, from not imposing enough structure, boundaries, and discipline.

Understanding and coming to terms with our own formative experiences is probably the most important psychological work any of us can do. It can be painful to peel away the denial that might have shielded us from some of the difficult realities, but this process is necessary to allow us to accept these truths. Acceptance then allows us to feel compassion for our younger selves, to acknowledge that as children we had little choice; we did our best; we couldn't have done otherwise. Then we can choose not to be victimized by these experiences. Instead of saying to ourselves "Why me?," we can ask ourselves, "What shall I do next?"

When we are thinking about what we shall do next, it is vital to remember that, no matter

> "Self-care is health care, nourishing you in this moment and nourishing the person you are becoming."
>
> **Suzy Reading, psychologist and author of *The Little Book of Self-Care***

what our earlier experiences have been, it is never too late to start to give ourselves what we lacked, to nurture and parent ourselves. We can do this through good self-care.

We can also achieve re-parenting (giving yourself what you didn't receive as a child) and re-nurturing through creativity and making things, and, if we are lucky, through our work. We can be restored through significant and positive relationships with friends and intimate relationships with our partners. It is never too late.

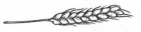

USING OUR IMPROVED SELF-KNOWLEDGE

I have found that some of my most helpful insights into what really matters to me have come in groups. In a group there are resonances and mirrorings that sometimes allow us to see ourselves with a clarity that more usually eludes us. Something can come straight up to the surface from a long way down.

After many years I was aware of a dissatisfaction with the work I was doing, a sense that what I was doing didn't really matter. I was fortunate enough to be part of a group and, on one particular occasion, I was pushed to say what I really cared about. With no sense of where the words were coming from, I blurted out, "I want people to know they are loved." Hearing myself saying these words out loud made me cry. I didn't know precisely what I meant, but I knew that this was profoundly true—this was what really mattered to me. As we've already seen, the way these things work is that we tend to be drawn to give others the thing we need ourselves. I have no doubt that a deep, unrequited need to be loved myself was the bottom line in question. However, it was a helpful revelation and the words stayed with me until eventually I made sense of them.

It took a long time for me to find the means to translate the sentiment into action and for it to influence decisions about how I spent my time and the sort of work I could do, but losing my job presented me with the chance to think carefully about what I wanted to do next. I decided to pause before jumping back into work. I realized that I wanted to do something creative, which helped people, and I didn't want to manage other people, but I couldn't work out what sort of job this might be. It was a friend's casual remark, "You should be doing something that involves talking" that, together with the remembered phrase about wanting people to know they are loved, somehow triggered in me the idea that training as a therapist would be what I would do.

As soon as I started my studies, I realized that listening was more important than speaking, but nevertheless, I felt I had found my niche. It does feel that this is what I do: I try to let people know they are valuable human beings worthy of love—in my role as a mother, as a therapist, as a baker of bread, and as a writer. I also am able to acknowledge where this drive comes from, and that is fine too. I use the word "try" because in my desire to have other people recognize their own worth, I have gotten it wrong sometimes and no doubt will continue to make mistakes in the future.

And I now see that I am doing what most of us do: we strive to give other people something we have needed ourselves. This is fine and a normal thing to happen. I have no doubt that my late parents loved me dearly, but it was not their way to show or say it.

The dynamic of being the oldest of six siblings, all close together in age, also meant that competing for attention was constant. Getting on with things, helping with the younger ones, and being responsible for myself was my way of getting parental approval. These circumstances meant that I grew up with a longing to know that I was loved, and a familiarity with looking after others. One of my challenges has been to learn to be able to look after myself too. My historic need to feel that I am loved has translated into a desire to give this reassurance to others. In choosing to train in therapy and indeed to opt for spending swathes of time baking bread to feed people, I was not at first conscious of what was going on beneath the surface. When we are unconsciously driven to do something, it just feels like a good idea. It is in retrospect and through being in a therapy group myself that I have started to make sense of it.

> Making bread and celebrating breadmaking and encouraging other people to discover the joys of making their own bread is part of my sense of purpose.

Whatever the unconscious processes, and whether we are aware of them or not, the important thing is if what we are being driven to do is in our own best interests. In a way, nothing matters more than this. Distinguishing between the destructive and self-limiting and the constructive and self-affirming is everything. The bottom line is that if we are behaving in a way that is destructive and self-limiting, whatever the reasons for this, change is desirable and possible. If we are tending to act in ways that are constructive and self-affirming, then again, regardless of the roots of this way of being, we are on the right road to further growth and fulfillment.

When we discover an element of our constructive and authentic purpose in life, it feels like coming home. If we then ask ourselves what values relate to this purpose, it all starts to make sense intellectually as well as emotionally. Making bread and celebrating breadmaking and encouraging other people to discover the joys of making their own bread is part of my sense of purpose. If I ask myself what values I have that mesh with breadmaking, these would be kindness and beauty. These things that I value translate into showing other people they are cared for or loved by giving them something nourishing, crafting something by hand, creating something with aesthetic value (because a loaf is beautiful even if it is imperfect), passing on the enthusiasm and skills to others, getting closer to nature, caring for the environment, and reminding us of the importance of slowing down and feeling grounded in these frantic times.

Some of these values and many others are shared and universal. Baking your own bread is an activity that can be an expression of your values too.

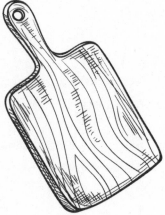

OTHER WAYS OF RECOGNIZING YOUR VALUES

Here are some of the ways that you can recognize your values. By asking yourself these questions and by mining your own preferences and passions, you can arrive at a list of the principles and beliefs that can be your guide to living authentically. This is not necessarily an easy process, especially if you feel you have spent a lot of time doing things that were not really "you." But another way of looking at this is that nothing is ever wasted and it is never too late to change direction. It is not unusual, when we start to understand ourselves better and make changes in our lives, to be faced with powerful feelings of sadness or regret that we didn't liberate ourselves in this way before. This is a time to exercise self-compassion and to accept that it is what it is; we did the best we could with what we knew at the time.

Asking yourself these questions will help you to identify what really matters to you, what you care passionately about.

What do you love talking about?

Left to your own devices, how do you choose to spend your time?

Is there anything you do in which you get so engrossed that you lose track of time?

What do you feel so strongly about that you get upset or angry about it?

**What do you want to make sure you
don't regret at the end of your days?**

(It is a truism, but nevertheless true, that no one, at the end of their
life, wishes they had spent more time in the office.)

**If you knew you only had a year to live,
how would you spend your time?**

**Who do you admire? Think of the qualities of your real,
historic, or fictional heroes and heroines. These are the
qualities that you value, that you already have, or need to
develop further in yourself. What are these qualities?**

Answering these questions will put you well on the road to being
able to know what really matters to you, which will throw light on
your sense of purpose, and in turn will present you with reasons for
getting up in the morning.

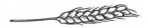

HAVING A SENSE OF PURPOSE

Dan Buettner is an author and researcher who has examined the
habits of populations across the globe that top longevity league
tables; he called these areas "blue zones." One of these blue zones
was Japan, in particular the occupants of the northern part of the
island of Okinawa. The people of Okinawa fare very well when it

comes to health and longevity. They live much longer than most of the rest of the world's population and they also suffer fewer illnesses, such as cancer and heart disease. Surveys of scientific research on longevity point to *ikigai,* the Japanese term for having a purpose in life, as well as diet, modest exercise, and forming strong social ties, as a key factor that unites all of the areas of the world where life expectancy is exceptionally high.

So, bringing together the identification of our own sense of purpose and values with how well this translates into our everyday decisions is pivotal to good mental health and could also have a significant impact on our physical health and longevity.

YOUR VALUES AND YOUR BREAD

Making decisions about the food that we buy and eat is something we probably do several times a day throughout our adult lives. Applying our values to these decisions contributes to the sense of integrity we feel when our actions agree with our beliefs. This connectedness between our ideals and what we choose to put on our plates then impacts our inner harmony. The growth of veganism is a good example of a food choice following on from a heartfelt belief.

How might our values impact on the way we get our hands on our daily bread? If we value the handmade, the unique, the highly nutritious, the delicious, the local, the sustainable, and the personal, then it would make perfect sense to make our own bread. If we choose to make our own bread, then what decisions might we make about the ingredients we make it with?

If you are making the effort to bake your own bread, then using the best-quality flour makes sense. Choosing to use organic, stone-ground flour from your nearest traditional mill will maximize the return from your effort by producing optimum taste and nourishment. You will also be supporting a local business and buying an unadulterated, quality product that has not traveled very far from field to mill to your oven.

Whatever sort of bread you make, good-quality flour will make a real difference. Making informed decisions about the food you eat, the sort of bread you choose to buy or bake, and the ingredients you choose to make it with can also make a real difference to your sense of self because it can be an expression of your beliefs and identity.

This connectedness between our ideals and what we choose to put on our plates then impacts our inner harmony.

We have looked at the lengthy process involved in making sourdough bread, but making a loaf of bread can be quick too. The following recipe is for soda bread and it can be whipped up in well under an hour from start to finish. Screens can gobble up our time, leaving us with nothing to show for it. Making a loaf of soda bread is time well spent and you still have the baking time to do something else.

When making this loaf, reflect on how your decision to bake bread is an expression of your values, what you think is important, and who you are.

Soda bread (with variations)

The only equipment you will need to make this bread is a mixing bowl, a spoon, and a baking sheet (lined with baking parchment to stop the bread from sticking). Soda bread relies on the chemical reaction of acid (from the buttermilk) with baking soda to produce the gas that raises the bread. This happens quickly, hence there's no need to knead or proof the dough. In fact it is best to avoid hanging around and get this loaf into the oven as soon as you have mixed it.

This recipe is for a whole-wheat version, but feel free to substitute all-purpose flour for some or all of the brown if you prefer a lighter loaf. You could bake it in a loaf pan but the traditional (Irish) way is to form a round loaf and to make a deep, cross-shaped cut in the dough. Apart from any symbolic significance, this helps the bread bake through thoroughly.

Makes 1 loaf

INGREDIENTS

4 cups (16 oz/450 g) whole-wheat flour, plus extra for dusting
   (or this loaf works well with a mixture of half white bread
   flour and half whole-wheat flour)
1 tsp fine salt (unrefined sea salt if possible)
1 tsp baking soda

1¾ cups (450 ml) buttermilk (or use milk with 1 tbsp lemon
   juice added to it)
splash of milk (optional—only if required)

METHOD

1. Heat the oven to 400°F/200°C.

2. Put the flour, salt, baking soda, and oats into a mixing
    bowl and stir. Make a dip or well in the center of the dry
    ingredients and stir in the buttermilk.

3. Transfer the dough to a lightly floured surface and
    use your hands to work it into a ball (it will be about
    6 inches in diameter). If it is too soft and sticky, add
    some flour. If it is too dry and not all the flour has been
    incorporated, add a splash of milk.

4. Put the ball of dough on the baking parchment on the
    baking sheet and cut a cross into the top. Cut into the
    dough quite deeply, about halfway down the depth of
    the loaf. It will immediately start to open up; this is fine
    and it is time to get it straight into the oven.

5. Bake for approximately 45 minutes or until the crust
    is browned and the loaf sounds hollow when tapped
    underneath.

6. Your soda bread can be cooled on a wire rack, but this is a bread that can also be eaten while it is still warm.

Reflect on how, in under an hour, you have produced a wholesome loaf of bread, an honest loaf, a rustic beauty, to share with people you care about.

There are hundreds of recipes for soda bread. Some recipes include a tablespoonful of molasses or honey, so try them out and see what you prefer. A lovely, savory version results from the addition of 4 oz (125 g) of grated hard cheese. A teatime, sweeter variation is to add 1 teaspoon of pie spice, ½ cup (100 g) of demerara sugar and 1 cup (150 g) of whatever dried fruit you have in the pantry (you could use raisins, currants, golden raisins, chopped dates, chopped dried apricots, or mixed peel).

This is a bread to make on impulse or when unexpected visitors arrive; it provides almost instant gratification. Why not invite a friend to enjoy it with you? Soda bread is best eaten on the day it is baked, so enjoy it while it is fresh. Soda bread goes wonderfully with butter and jam or marmalade but also with cheese or soups or stews (especially Irish stew).

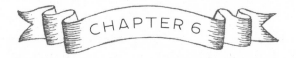

CHAPTER 6

Accepting Imperfection

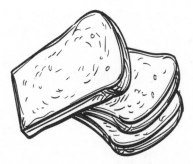

Loaves like bricks; loaves welded to their pans; loaves sunken on top; wildly split; raw in the middle; soggy on the bottom; burned; strange-tasting; flat as pancakes; too dry; too crumbly; impossible to slice. I could go on. These are just some of the many things that have gone wrong for me while baking bread. It is true that I might feel slight annoyance or disappointment if a loaf doesn't turn out as well as I'd hoped it would, but I have learned to accept the mishaps as helpful evidence of my fallibility and the fact that there are many variables that are beyond my control. You may have already discovered for yourself that things can go wrong, that breadmaking is not an exact science, that your loaves sometimes don't turn out as expected. The fact that making bread can be unpredictable and prone to misfortune means that it has the potential to present us with reminders of our own flaws and weaknesses. It also offers us regular prompts to remember the tendency of the world to present us with the unexpected and unwelcome. This is a good thing. Like a Roman general with a slave whispering in his ear that he is mortal, being a bread baker means that you will be regularly reminded of your imperfection and impermanence.

DEALING WITH REAL ADVERSITY

Learning to accept what is real and to refrain from beating ourselves up when something minor goes wrong—like a loaf collapsing—is a meditation and a preparation. It is a way of developing the capacity to accept and go beyond suffering and hardship when something really important does go wrong. I am thinking of those life events that we can do nothing about. This does not mean that we should deny our emotional reality—the emotional pain we can experience when life deals us a difficult challenge. On the contrary, part of the art of acceptance is to accept the reality of what we are feeling, as well as the reality of what has happened; to allow ourselves to feel what we are feeling, however painful. It is only by going through these feelings that we can process what has happened to us or what has happened to the people we love. There is no escape, only delay. If we try to stop ourselves feeling, then the unexpressed emotions tend to persist, often in the form of physical or mental ill health. By accepting and experiencing the reality of what has happened to us, and the validity and strength of our emotional responses, we can find ways of adjusting to what has come about. We adapt to the new normal. We find a way to carry on.

This is what we know about what works when we are faced with difficult life events. The extremes of reaction don't work very well at all.

The first extreme is denial, parceling away the actuality of what is happening or has happened and carrying on as normal (or more realistically, trying to carry on as normal). Fear of uncontrollable or unbearable emotion often fuels this approach and the feelings are habitually bundled away with the truth. This response to trauma or distressing events buys us temporary relief and is understandable, but it is not sustainable. The feelings that have been repressed or suppressed don't go away and they can emerge later in other forms. Classic examples of this are depression resulting from unexpressed grief, or sadness and anxiety as a product of unexpressed anger.

> We can find ways of adjusting to what has come about. We adapt to the new normal. We find a way to carry on.

The other extreme is not helpful either. If we focus exclusively on what has happened, becoming obsessed with difficult life events in such a way that we can't actually function, we can become stuck. This pattern is characterized by rumination, going over and over what has happened. This circular thinking doesn't get us anywhere: "Why has this happened?" or "Why me?" keep us trapped, unable to move on.

As so often is the case, the middle way is what allows us to move forward, to process what has happened both intellectually and emotionally. We need to be able to accept, feel, think, and talk about what has happened. By facing the reality and feeling the emotions, by processing through thought and words, we can move through the experience and, in time, eventually move on from it. This is different from forgetting or blanking out, it is a way of making sense of what has happened in such a way that we can carry on to the future.

The better we have become at the art of acceptance, then the more likely we are to be able to accept the reality of the distressing situations we or people we care about are in. Importantly, this does not mean we have to like whatever it is that is distressing us, or indeed the feelings that go with it. A helpful mantra to adopt is: "*It is what it is.*"

THE ART OF ACCEPTANCE

Teaching ourselves the art of acceptance is something that can be a lifelong enterprise and it can be one of the most liberating and healing lessons we can give ourselves. We can practice it every day and baking bread gives us that opportunity. Practicing with small things, like baking bread, makes it easier to summon up acceptance and calm when bigger things go wrong. This all matters because if we develop the ability to accept the reality of what is happening, and how we feel about it, then we are less likely to fall into the trap of denial. If we can accept the reality we are in and the emotions we are feeling, no matter how distressing, we are more likely to be able to talk to other people, seek support, and process our experiences.

I hadn't learned about the importance of acceptance when I

faced adversity at the end of my teens. I was a 19-year-old psychology student when I became pregnant with my first daughter. I got married and was still 19 when she was born prematurely with serious neurological problems. Looking back, it was traumatic for all three of us. At the time, I was so desperate to prove to everyone that I could be a good, responsible mother that I buried my emotions. I took a sideways step from a student life of essays and alcohol into a parallel universe of hospital appointments, operations, and anxiety. I did need to get on with it, which is what happened, but I didn't need to deny my feelings in the way that I did. I think as a consequence, I dipped in and out of low mood for a number of years, but I was adept at hiding it.

I have a clear memory of a small, domestic incident that crystallizes that time for me. We had a Minton china bowl. I thought it was the most beautiful object I had ever owned. Translucent white with delicate painted flowers, it sat on a shelf and somehow I knocked it off. It broke cleanly into two pieces. I wept for hours. I think now, in weeping so copiously for the cracked bowl, I was shedding tears for my child and for myself. I think I thought I was broken too. Again, looking back, the bowl would have been easy to mend. Instead I can remember with absolute clarity my train of thought at that time. It included the belief that there would never be a moment when I would have the energy to buy glue or would have the time to hold the two severed halves together until they stuck. I just gazed at the broken china lying against potato peelings in the trash and cried.

I loved and love my daughter utterly, as I do all my now grown-up

By learning to be tolerant of small things going wrong, we are teaching ourselves skills that will mean we are better placed to weather the bigger storms that may come our way.

children. I wonder if part of me felt I would have been somehow disloyal to her, and my love for her, if I had acknowledged my own sense of loss. It was only decades later that I was able to see, possibly for the first time, how desperately difficult an experience this all must have been for an adolescent who was needy herself. Back then I only allowed myself occasional, private moments of mourning for how I imagined my daughter might have been without the brain damage. It strikes me now that I didn't register the loss of the more carefree, early adult years I might have expected to have. Of course, everything was not tragic at that time, there were good things in my life happening too. It was just that the enormity of what had happened to my first daughter was woven through everything I experienced.

There is a school of thinking which holds that normal, sane mental functioning is predicated on a sort of charmed existence. The thesis is that we can go on being cheerful and positive because we are in healthy denial about existential realities such as illness, accidents, and mortality. The theory suggests that if we were to spend our days fully aware of the likelihood of the disasters lurking around every corner, then we would indeed be depressed and would probably never make it out of bed in the morning. Like most of us, I operated according to the unspoken assumption that serious ill health, car crashes, fires, or earthquakes happened to other people. Then, when something extremely challenging did happen, the rug was completely pulled out from under this assumption. If this can go wrong, then anything can go wrong, I thought. It took me a long time to rebuild anything resembling optimism. I can remember back then, thinking that I would probably never be happy again: that whatever wonderful, new thing materialized, it would always be somehow marred by remembering what had already happened.

I was wrong.

Wonderful things have happened: adored new babies, relationships, studies, fulfilling work, and I have experienced them all (at times) with unadulterated joy. Rather than becoming a permanent stain on happiness, my daughter's struggles have become part of who I am as well as part of who she is. When my daughter was a little older, a friend said something that had a profound impact on me. He said: "I wouldn't want her to be any different, we love her; she's fine the way she is." I think it was a pivotal moment, prompting me to move toward acceptance and the future.

I am not for a minute equating serious life events with bread-baking adversities, or—what would be even more absurd—disability with imperfect loaves. What I do want to convey is the fundamental truth that we are all imperfect and that there is beauty in our differences and individualities. It is also true that our resilience and ability to bounce back from challenges is something that we can get better at; that we can work at; that we can grow. By learning to be tolerant of small things going wrong, as we have ample opportunity to do when we are baking bread, then we are teaching ourselves skills that will mean we are better placed to weather the bigger storms that may come our way. None of us can ever gain immunity from suffering, but we can learn to make it easier for ourselves to recover from it.

Using our breadmaking as a way of developing the art of acceptance, especially when things do not turn out as expected, is one of the ways we can build it into a habit. The habit of acceptance is something which enables us to deal better with real adversity.

KINTSUGI: CELEBRATING IMPERFECTION

When I was despairing about my broken bowl and everything it symbolized, the idea that being broken was not a permanent state was something I couldn't compute. I knew in theory that things could be mended, but somehow I didn't believe it applied to me. I felt that once something was broken, that was it, "All the king's horses and all the king's men, couldn't put Humpty together again." Being broken meant being spoiled, irrevocably spoiled. I heard childhood admonitions echoing, "You've done it now," "It's all ruined," "You stupid girl."

Even as a child, I think I had an inkling that there was something not right about being shamed for breaking or losing something you actually loved. It took a long time before I realized that breaking things, making mistakes, and doing things you later regretted was normal. Everyone does it. It is part of being human and, what is more, it is possible to be alright again; broken things can be mended and healed; recovery is possible. Making mistakes didn't mean your life was ruined, it meant you were normal. Understanding these things, which I realize are blatantly obvious to some people, paved the way for me to start to show myself some compassion, to stop giving myself the hard time I had internalized from the past. And then it gets even better.

Kintsugi is the Japanese art of mending broken pottery with seams of precious metals, with gold or silver. I hadn't heard of kintsugi back then, or its potential to transform damaged china in this incredible way. Maybe the idea would have been so far removed from my mindset that I wouldn't have been able to register it, either as a literal way to mend my bowl or as a symbol of how I too could be fixed. In both cases it would have been exactly what I needed to hear. It is a transformative concept. The opposite of invisible mending, it is making a feature of something having been smashed. It is the broken object becoming better than new; celebrating the fact that something has been broken and literally highlighting the cracks. It is an impressive approach when it comes to fixing broken ceramics, but it is an even more potent metaphor and guide for how we can deal with our emotional scars. We have all experienced suffering or emotional pain in different ways, but what can unite us is the fact that we have found a way of surviving, we are here.

The emotional scars we carry are nothing to be ashamed of; they are not to be hidden away—they can be gilded and celebrated. The powerful influence of this approach is evident now in the growing number of mental health campaigners who have chosen to reveal their own emotional scars and in doing so have inspired many others to experience the liberation that acceptance brings about.

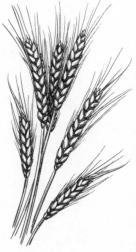

Having suffered, having been hurt, having been let down by people we should have been able to rely on, having experienced neglect, abandonment, or abuse—it is important to remember that none of these things are signs of weakness or are anything to feel shame about. Yes, we are left with mental scars, but we can choose to see these scars as marks of our survival. We can remind ourselves:

I did nothing wrong.

I did the best I could.

I couldn't have done it differently.

We can polish up our scars. We can honor the marks of what we have survived and metaphorically gild them.

Decades since it was consigned to landfill, in my mind's eye I can still see that delicate bowl I broke, and I can imagine it now, joined back together with a thick vein of gold. It seems I have carried it with me for all of these years and now maybe it has eventually served its purpose in me telling its story.

BREAKING THE CHAIN REACTION

Understanding and accepting the inevitability of imperfection is another piece of psychological learning that could liberate you from some forms of anxiety and low mood.

This is quite a claim, but it rests on the nature of emotional chain reactions—the way one psychological problem can lead to another. There is one particular sequence that presents itself often; this is:

low self-esteem, leading to

perfectionism, leading to

anxiety, leading to

low mood, and then back around to

further low self-esteem

Sometimes when we are not responsive to therapy or self-help treatments for anxiety or low mood, it is because we have not identified what lies behind them and we need help from therapy to do this work—to see past the blind spots about ourselves. In my work with young people, one of the most common underlying issues is a pair of difficulties that tend to co-exist. These are low self-esteem and then the perfectionist tendencies we develop to compensate for it. Working on these underlying problems of low self-esteem and perfectionism often has a significant, beneficial impact on anxiety or low mood. The stronger our sense of our own intrinsic worth, the less reliant we become on what other people think about us, or in proving ourselves through our achievements. This then takes away, or considerably dilutes, any worries we have about how we are perceived or about our success or lack of it.

LOW SELF-ESTEEM: IF I DO SOMETHING WRONG
I WILL BE JUDGED

Low self-esteem leads us to self-limiting, self-critical, and self-sabotaging behaviors which then reinforce our negative self-appraisals. One of the powerful, inner forces that can stop us from exploring, trying new things, and experimenting, is the fear of making mistakes or the fear of failure. This is something we all experience to varying degrees, but what fear of making mistakes or fear of failure usually comes down to is fear of being negatively judged. This fear is especially dominant if we associate being negatively judged with being rejected or abandoned.

We tend to fear the things that have already happened to us. If we fear being judged, we probably experienced being judged harshly when we were younger. If you can imagine the opposite, a childhood where making mistakes or failing resulted in empathy, acceptance, love, and encouragement to keep trying, then you might start to see how the problem isn't making mistakes per se, but rather the way our attitude toward making mistakes has been shaped. If we have had repeated experiences of being put down or condemned for making errors, then we are likely to have internalized these critical voices. We will then limit ourselves and our ambitions. We will have a tendency

The answer is not to continue to avoid situations or activities where we fear we will be criticized, but to build up a positive sense of self-worth by doing it anyway.

to "play it safe" to try to minimize the risk of being disapproved of or criticized. This sort of avoidance can quickly become a habit. The more we avoid doing anything new, anything we might not be very good at to begin with (actually, that is most things we haven't tried before), the more established the pattern of avoidance becomes and the harder it is to break it. There is a price we pay in these situations where we fear that we could be judged. If we try to buy ourselves protection from disapproval or criticism by not writing the book, not saying what we really think, not applying for the promotion, not going to the party, not singing the solo, not baking the loaf, then we might feel safe in the short term, but we are incurring a high penalty for this apparent escape from judgement. We are limiting ourselves and our lives unnecessarily. We are hobbling ourselves and not giving ourselves the chance to realize that actually, we could do these things. Low self-esteem means we tend to consistently underestimate our own strengths and abilities, further encouraging us to give up before we even start.

Even if we couldn't do whatever it is we are afraid of failing at, we probably wouldn't be judged anyway. And if we were judged, so what? The criticism tells us more about the person who feels the need to disparage others than it ever says about us.

The answer is not to continue to avoid situations or activities where we fear we will be criticized, but to build up a positive sense of self-worth by doing it anyway. With higher self-esteem, we are less dependent on the approval of others and therefore less fearful of doing things that might not go well at first.

Ask yourself if there is anything you have not done because of fear that you would not be good enough, or fear of disapproval, or fear of judgement. What step could you take now that would put you on the road to doing that thing you avoided?

Often it is behavioral change that will allow us to step sideways from the vicious circle of low self-esteem and avoidance. The sideward move takes us to a virtuous circle where daring to do something we are afraid of (that we are avoiding for reasons of feared disapproval) offers us the chance to experience success and, at the very least, gives us evidence of the fact that we have tried. All this makes us feel better about ourselves. This in turn builds our confidence and self-esteem and makes it more likely that we will try something else that scares us in the future.

PERFECTIONISM: IF I DO EVERYTHING PERFECTLY I CAN'T BE JUDGED

If we have low self-esteem then we tend to try to compensate for this lack of faith in our own inherent worth by choosing some external form of validation to allow us to feel okay. For many people it is academic, career, or financial success they will use as a way of feeling positive about themselves; for others, their perfectionist rules are related to their appearance or popularity. These qualifications are all characterized by being contingent on something external to the self, which is not amenable to control. Someone would effectively be saying to themselves, for example: "As long as I get top grades for my essays or a promotion at work then I must be alright." Someone with this perfectionist rule will feel fine about themselves for as long as their grades keep them at the top of the class, or they are offered a better job. But as soon as, for whatever reason, the grades are no longer the best, or they are passed over for promotion, this person will not only react with normal disappointment but will be devastated by having their reason for feeling good about themselves taken away.

Perfectionist rules and assumptions are many and varied but here are some more examples:

- I must never offend anybody

- I must always be thin

- I must never be late

- I must always have a partner

- I must always do the right thing

- I must never show my feelings

- I must always appear to be happy

- I must always look perfect

- I must always be fun to be with

- I have to be popular

- I have to have lots of friends

- I must never make mistakes

- I must always appear to be clever

- I must never appear anxious

- I must ensure that everyone around me is happy

- ❧ I must never look foolish

- ❧ I must always have something witty to say

- ❧ I must be good at everything

- ❧ I must never upset anyone

- ❧ I must earn a lot of money

- ❧ I must always win at sports

- ❧ I must always take care of everyone else

These and all other perfectionist rules are characterized by being unreasonable and unhelpful. They can lead to anxiety because of the precariousness of this sort of contingent self-worth. If your reason for feeling okay about yourself is something outside your own direct control, then worry and fear about your rules not being met can become chronic. It is as if you are living on the edge of disaster all the time. The feared calamity would be being exposed as imperfect, not good enough.

This anxiety can have a direct, negative impact on performance, actually making it more likely that someone will make a mistake, for example, through nervousness. The anxiety also leads to people trying too hard to meet their unrealistic goals, again this can lead to unintended consequences. An example might be someone who has a perfectionist rule that they must be liked by everyone. Such a rule will inevitably lead this person to try too hard to please and ingratiate themselves with others. The result of this effort, paradoxically, is usually to put people off. Sensing the discomfort of others in their presence, the person trying too hard will have their underlying low self-esteem reinforced and their mood will drop.

We all need rules, assumptions, and beliefs to operate, but there is a big difference between helpful rules and unhelpful rules. Perfectionist rules are particularly unhelpful because they are characterized by not being reliably achievable. Consider the difference between "I must always be the best," and "I will always try my best."

Trying your best is something you can consciously choose to do and could conceivably achieve. Always being the best is setting yourself up for anxiety and failure. Being the best in the class, company, competition, family is beyond your control. This is, as you will know, because you cannot determine variables, such as what other people do.

So, a helpful step toward overcoming a tendency to perfectionism is to recognize when you are operating according to a perfectionist rule. If you realize you are worried or anxious about something, it is really helpful to ask yourself whether or not you are using one of these unhelpful rules. If you are, then the good news, again, is that you can change it. We can consciously adjust the rule to morph it into a more balanced version of itself, a version that is reasonable and achievable. An example would be to shift from: "I must never upset anyone," to, "I don't set out to upset anyone, but sometimes it is beyond my control and it doesn't make me a bad person if it happens."

Or, from: "I must always have a partner," to "Being in a relationship can be great but I do not need to have a partner to be acceptable as a person."

Try to work on more balanced and helpful versions of the examples of perfectionist rules and assumptions, and perhaps also ones you have identified that you use yourself. If you are feeling anxious about a situation, ask yourself:

Am I using a perfectionist rule here?

If I am, what is it?

What would be a more reasonable version of this rule?

A common perfectionist belief is the conviction that we must be able to do something very well, right away. If we think there is a chance that we will fail or do something badly when we first try to speak French, ski, bake a loaf of bread, or write a poem, then chances are we are unlikely to try these things or take chances with our learning. The reality is that to progress up any learning curve, we need to be able to tolerate doing badly at first, then through practicing we will improve. If we cannot tolerate initial incompetence then we are unlikely to ever try and repeat things that could expand and enrich our lives. Paradoxically, this in turn reinforces our negative self-view—we will see ourselves as someone who can't speak French, ski, bake bread, or write poetry. Whereas if we can challenge the perfectionist beliefs, we can tolerate making mistakes and messing up at the beginning so that we can get on to the learning curve that will allow us to see ourselves as triers and achievers. This is why it is so important to praise children for effort, for trying, and for perseverance, not just for results or talent.

The acceptance of impermanence reminds us that nothing lasts forever and therefore we should value every day we have on this earth as well as the loaves we make.

Because making bread can present us with setbacks, things not going according to plan, we can actually use it as a conscious exercise in teaching ourselves to let go of perfectionist expectations. By giving ourselves the chance to learn to better tolerate baking mistakes or unintended results, we can prepare ourselves to spread this attitude beyond breadmaking into our wider lives and reap considerable psychological rewards.

IMPERFECT AND IMPERMANENT

The Japanese concept of *wabi-sabi* celebrates the beauty of imperfection and qualities of impermanence and both are exemplified in bread and breadmaking. The imperfect loaf stands for the imperfect life that we all lead.

In learning to accept imperfection in our loaves, we can learn to accept it in our lives too. The acceptance of imperfection allows us to develop compassion for ourselves, to be kinder to ourselves, and to worry less. The acceptance of impermanence reminds us that nothing lasts forever and that therefore we should value every day we have on this earth as well as the loaves we make.

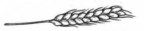

TECHNIQUES AND RECIPES FOR NEVER WASTING A CRUMB

Whatever sort of bread you make and no matter how "imperfect" it is, it is precious. You will not want to waste a single slice, and this is exactly how it should be. Food waste is a problem of colossal proportion and reducing it needs to be a priority for us all. When you have made something yourself from scratch, you value it properly.

Despite not having the preservatives that are added to factory-made bread, sourdough loaves can still be edible a week after baking. Bread that is made more rapidly, such as soda bread, will start to go stale after a day; but there is always a way of using up any sort of homemade bread and avoiding waste.

It may well be that you, your family, and friends are so enamored of the bread you make that there is never any left over, but there may be occasions when you have more bread than there are mouths to feed at the time, or maybe your loaf is starting to go a bit dry or stale before you can get through it. In his book *Do Sourdough: Slow Bread for Busy Lives*, Andrew Whitley proposes "The Seven Days of Bread" with ideas for uses of bread as it hardens and dries over a week. I don't think this list can be bettered. As well as eating it fresh and then making sandwiches, he suggests toast, bruschetta, making crispbreads, croutons, and finally breadcrumbs as great ways to make use of bread as it ages.

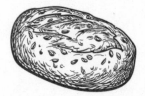

Toast can be made from bread that is past its springy best. Dense, whole-grain bread can hold a lot of heat when toasted, so give it time to cool down to make sure that you don't burn your mouth.

Bruschetta made from homemade bread is delicious. It works very well when the bread is turning stale and is already a bit dry, as it needs less toasting, holds its shape, and soaks up the oil. After lightly toasting the bread, top it with a drizzle of olive oil and salad leaves, tomatoes, goat cheese, or olives.

Crispbreads can be made from very thinly sliced, hardening bread that is then dried out further on a baking sheet in the oven at a low temperature—275°F/140°C. The idea is to make them crisp without browning them. They are being dried rather than baked, and this can take up to an hour (depending on how thinly you have managed to slice the bread). The crispbreads that result keep well in an airtight tin for at least another week and could mean that you never need to buy expensive crackers for cheese again. They are also great for pâté or for eating with hummus or other dips.

Croutons are a good addition to soup or salads. Make them by cutting old bread into cubes and then frying these in olive oil over a medium heat until they turn golden.

Breadcrumbs can be made from whatever odds and ends of bread you have. Breadcrumbs are made by crumbling the bread between your fingers or by using a food processor—the latter can be a good way of breaking down crusts in particular. Fresh breadcrumbs (although made with stale bread) can be used to thicken other dishes or as an ingredient in sauces. They won't keep for more than a day or two, so if you want to keep them for longer, drying them out is the answer. Place them on a baking sheet in a low oven (275°F/140°C) for about an hour, until dry and crisp but not browned, and then keep them in an airtight container for up to three months. Dried breadcrumbs can be used for coating foods before frying or as a topping. As well as being used when they are freshly made or dried, breadcrumbs can also be frozen in either state in a freezer bag.

Freezing homemade bread works well in any form: whole, sliced, diced, or crumbed. An efficient way to freeze leftover bread you know you won't eat right away is to slice the bread and then freeze it in an airtight container or a reusable, resealable freezer bag. This way you can take out of the freezer exactly what you need, slice by slice, and it can be toasted straight from frozen. If you have deliberately made extra bread for the freezer, then freezing it whole as soon as it has cooled will preserve its quality.

Apple Brown Betty

This recipe is a wonderful way to use slices of bread that are past their best, but still more than edible. Apple Brown Betty has traditionally been made on both sides of the Atlantic. It is a baked dessert made up of layers of buttered bread and fruit sweetened with syrup or brown sugar. There are variations that use breadcrumbs mixed with melted butter, but this version is made from slices of stale bread and is adapted from a Constance Spry recipe. It provides yet another level of transformation for this treasured commodity of homemade bread.

You will need an ovenproof dish—a deepish, oval pie dish would be ideal. There are not precise quantities for this recipe, it is a matter of matching the size of the dish to the amount of bread and apples you have available or vice versa. If you were using six slices of bread, for example, then four dessert apples or two larger cooking apples would be about right and this would serve four. The dessert can also be made with other fruits, such as plums, blackberries, or gooseberries, either on their own or mixed with apples. Nothing bad will happen if you use more fruit than this or if you need to use more bread and fruit to fill your dish; you will just need to increase the amount of sugar or syrup accordingly.

INGREDIENTS

*sliced, stale bread (hard crusts removed—they can be used to
   make breadcrumbs)*
butter (enough to butter the bread on both sides)
apples, peeled, cored, and thinly sliced
brown sugar, golden syrup, or maple syrup

METHOD

1. Heat the oven to 375°F/190°C.

2. Generously butter the slices of bread on both sides and
   cut each slice into quarters.

3. Cover the bottom of the ovenproof dish with a single,
   slightly overlapping layer of bread.

4. Cover this with a layer of the apple slices—this should
   be two or three slices deep.

5. Sprinkle the fruit with a good tablespoon of brown
   sugar or syrup.

6. Cover the layer of fruit with another layer of bread.

7. Now add the rest of the apple slices and again sweeten
   with a good tablespoon of sugar or syrup.

8. Lastly, arrange the remaining bread so that it covers the surface of the fruit and add a final tablespoon of sugar or syrup.

9. Bake for 30–40 minutes, until brown on the top and a knife will go straight through to the bottom of the dish, indicating that the apples are soft.

Whichever fruit you have used, this is a great dessert, served warm, straight from the dish, with ice cream, cream, or custard, and you will have made something that has helped prevent good food going to waste, your cherished bread. Reflect on how, by making this dessert, you are making a small step in the collective journey of reducing the amount of food waste produced on the planet. Whatever it looks like, celebrate your dessert's perfect imperfections and accept and enjoy it just the way it is.

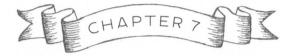

CHAPTER 7

Connecting with Others

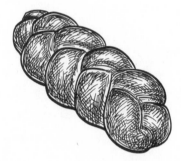

We had gotten as far as Heathrow and I still didn't know where my new husband was taking me for our honeymoon; this had not been helpful when packing. There was one name on the departure board that I wasn't familiar with, Yerevan. My uneasiness about surprises turned to pleasure and curiosity when I realized that Yerevan, the capital of Armenia, was indeed where we were going.

It was late at night when we arrived. We were met by an interpreter who handed me a bunch of lilies of the valley so large it took both hands to hold them. Flowers were important in Armenia. We drove past lightbulb-lit stalls selling gorgeous bouquets and wine at one o'clock in the morning. This was a strong indication of the sort of place we had come to.

Hospitality was almost embarrassingly generous. This was at the end of the 1990s and, confirming a universal paradox, it was people who were not at all wealthy who were so warmly giving and kind. Wherever we sat down to eat or drink, the wonderful wine was accompanied by elaborate toasts to our health and to Bobby Charlton and Winston Churchill. We were repeatedly invited to join strangers at restaurant tables and picnics outside monasteries to share their food.

The natural cordiality in this part of the world is boosted by the belief that guests are sent by God. To treat your visitors with kindness is to expect happiness to come back to your own household; there must have been many happy houses after our visit. We feasted on yogurt, great handfuls of unidentified herbs, and soft cheese wrapped in lavash. A staple flatbread made in clay ovens sunk into the ground, lavash was everywhere. We watched the breads being made by small teams of women: one making smooth balls of the simple flour and water dough, another rolling them out with a thin rolling pin to the exact size for another to

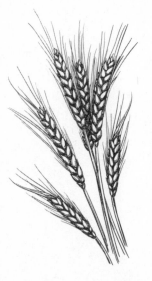

stretch the thin sheet of dough over a cushioned oval about 2 feet long that looked like a little ironing board. The last woman in the baking chain bent down and slapped the thin dough on its pad against the hot wall of the oven, where it blistered and bubbled for about half a minute before being expertly hooked out, somehow never dropping to the fire at the bottom of the pit.

We were invited to a riverside barbecue where the lavash was made by the women and the men cooked meat over the open fire. Knowing we were just married, our new friends insisted we enact a ritual to ensure our future prosperity, fertility, and health. Standing together, a lavash was draped over each of our shoulders. We then had to break china plates by stamping on them. This accomplished, it meant that we would never go hungry and that this would be the last thing broken in our marriage. It was an auspicious start to our life together. Bread was our symbol of love and connection and we were honeymooning in a country where bread is eaten with every meal and is treated, as is so rightly deserved, as a national treasure.

THE UNIVERSAL CULTURE OF BREADMAKING

In Armenia, bread is not just central to the cuisine, it is at the heart of the culture, both in the way it is made and in the way it is shared. In 2014, UNESCO added Armenian lavash to its List of the Intangible Cultural Heritage of Humanity. Bread plays a central role in rituals and in everyday life all over the world. It is very difficult to identify any parts of the world where bread is not eaten and where it does not hold some religious or cultural significance. Bread is part of our identities; the making and sharing of bread is symbolic of nurture, of fertility. Across the globe, as in Armenia, traditionally women are often the bread bakers; the origins of the word "lady" lie in the old English for "kneader of dough."

But breadmaking is for everyone, regardless of gender. Some of the most important pioneers of real bread-baking and the resurgence of sourdough bread, for example, are men. Teaching our boys to cook and bake has happily become normal. It is almost as if baking bread is in our collective memories. When one of my sons, a soldier, was on active duty a long way from home, he improvised a bread oven, building it using a metal cartridge box. He baked bread for the men in his section, providing comfort as well as nourishment. The urge to make bread is universal. Bread stands for home and making it can provide solace. It is telling that the first businesses to spring up in refugee camps are usually bakeries.

Bread is everywhere and everywhere it is different. Across Asia there are thousands of regional variations, from *mantou* (steamed buns) in the north of China to naan, roti, chapattis, and paratha across India. Rather than being baked on a griddle or in a tandoor, in Kazakhstan the bread is baked at home in a mini oven made of two heavy metal pans over an open fire. Historically the Kazakhs were a nomadic people and the practice of using a portable oven has persisted, sometimes using an open fire, sometimes on an electric stove.

Moving north, in Sweden breadmaking can involve the whole family, from grandparents to young children. Speaking about the special role of bread in Nordic culture, the acclaimed chef Magnus Nilsson talks about the breaking and sharing of bread as a "communal, ritual act," and says that in Christian significance, bread is so important that it can be compared to the gift of children. He describes how the making, as well as the eating, of bread can also be a group activity. Twice a year in parts of Sweden, extended families come together to batch bake large quantities of flatbreads that they will leave to dry and will then last them for months. He describes his family doing this and baking hundreds of flatbreads a day in a big wood-fired oven. Baking bread can connect people and the eating of bread as a collective act is something that contributes to our sense of belonging and connection to others.

In Africa, we find a huge variety of breads across the continent. Injera is a spongy, sourdough flatbread that is a daily staple in Ethiopia and Eritrea and has been for thousands of years. It is made from a mixture of ground teff seeds and water, which is left to ferment over a few days into a thin paste, then poured on to and baked on a large heated griddle. This large, flat bread then becomes the

The urge to make bread is universal. Bread stands for home and making it can provide solace.

shared tablecloth, plate, and eating utensils for the people sharing a meal. Stews and salads and extra injera are piled on top of the wide injera base and the juices soak into the bread. Everyone uses the bread to scoop up the other foods and then eats the base injera, which is rich with the delicious sauces from the stews. When the meal is over, there is no waste (and no dishes to wash).

Native American pueblo bread is baked in the southwest United States and in some parts of South America. The women of the community bake the bread using an outdoor oven that is shaped like a beehive and made of layers of straw and clay. It is heated with a fire made from piñon wood. Bread is baked in large batches to feed families or to sell.

Indigenous people in Australia had a long tradition of making bread from ground seeds, called bush bread or seed cakes. This bread was high in protein as well as carbohydrates. Again it was the women who collected and prepared the seeds, grinding them

There is a representation of our common humanity in the breaking, tearing, or cutting of a loaf of bread. It is hard to be the enemy of someone you have broken bread with.

into flour and baking bread in the embers of open fires. The arrival of processed white flour led to the decline of traditional seed bread, though there is still a tradition of baking bread in the embers of a fire, which is called "damper."

Whether we use open fires or modern ovens, baking bread connects us directly with our ancestors and our global brothers and sisters. The instinct to make, eat, and share bread is a very deep one and a universal one.

THE NEED FOR BELONGING

It is ironic that now we are so digitally entwined and connected, loneliness has simultaneously increased as a problem across all age groups. We are starting to recognize that online connection is not a substitute for human contact and being together. We are social creatures; we exist in relationship to others.

This need for a sense of belonging is in all of us. It is a fundamental driver and the absence of it can lead to isolation, emotional distress, a lack of purpose, and physical and mental health problems. The evidence from parts of the world with the greatest longevity, such as Okinawa in Japan (for more on this see also page 124), points to membership of groups and supportive relationships as a key factor in living a long and healthy life. On this Japanese island where there is a high number of healthy centenarians, people tend to grow up and then stay living in the same place. In childhood, groups of children are allocated to a *moai*—or friendship—group. The groups of five or six children then stick together for life, providing each other with a social and emotional safety net. If we can be part of a community and have a meaningful role in it, this means that we care about it, and it cares about us. This provides a tremendous protection against purposelessness, low mood, and anxiety.

There is a representation of our common humanity in the breaking, tearing, or cutting of a loaf of bread and it being shared around the table, everyone eating a part of the same whole. The sharing of the bread embodies the feeling of belonging. It is hard to be the enemy of someone you have broken bread with.

The need to belong, the need to feel we are part of something, to know that there is a place for us among others is everywhere. And so is bread. Bringing these two universals together, our need for belonging and the making of bread presents us with wonderful opportunities to connect with others.

BREAD CONNECTING COMMUNITIES

The Real Bread Campaign, based in the UK, is one of a number of organizations around the world that supports the baking of real bread (bread made without the use of processing aids or any other artificial additives). As well as promoting the interests of professional and home bakers of real bread, it also promotes social enterprises and local projects that use bread-baking as a means to improve lives and connect communities. There are baking projects in prisons and for ex-offenders; with people who have learning disabilities; for people struggling with their mental or physical health; for youth groups, refugees, veterans of the armed forces, children, and for people living with dementia. There are community bakeries that encourage the involvement of local people and that offer training opportunities to people who are out of work or socially excluded.

The ancient tradition of community bread ovens in public places is also being revived with numerous examples springing up, particularly in the U.S. There are some parts of the world, such as in Morocco, where this traditional and communal approach to baking bread has never gone away. There, even when people have ovens in their own houses, it is still normal to take bread to a communal, community oven to bake.

Bread Is Gold is the name of a book of inspiring recipes compiled by the Italian chef Massimo Bottura, who is also dedicated to fighting food waste. The title started with a remembered childhood dessert made of leftover bread, milk, and sugar, but it became something much bigger. *Bread Is Gold* became the rallying cry for initiatives to use food that would otherwise go to waste and to give it to people who needed it most. Bottura believed in the importance of beauty as well as kindness, and the refectory he set up in a rundown area of Milan—Refettorio Ambrosiano—was created in an abandoned building that was transformed by architects and 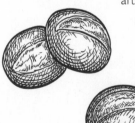 artists into a beautiful space. Likewise, the food that was imperfect—past its sell-by date or damaged in some way—was transformed by his chefs and volunteers into delicious and proper dishes for the guests who came from local shelters for homeless people. It is the essence of the Refettorio that the guests are all treated with dignity and respect. They are welcomed into a beautiful dining room and given a wonderful meal.

The project is still running and Bottura and his wife, Lara Gilmore, have set up an international movement called Food for Soul, to support similar projects worldwide, based on the premise that cooking is an act of love. There are refectories in Italy, France, England, and Brazil, with plans for more in other countries. The refectories serve food to vulnerable guests five days a week. "Social tables," another Food for Soul initiative, involves a meal being served in another community venue once a week with the same adherence to the principles of kindness, quality, and beauty.

YOU: CONNECTING THROUGH BREAD

My hope in writing this book has been to provide you with inspiration, a set of really compelling reasons, and the information you need to start baking your own bread. I want you to share the pleasure and sense of satisfaction that can come from learning a craft, such as breadmaking, and producing something beautiful and nourishing with your own hands. I want you to experience the wonder of transforming flour, water, and salt into flavorful, crusty loaves. I think that baking bread can be an act of love and I want to give this to you.

It need not stop with you, though. The final gift of breadmaking is to spread the word, for you to express your care for others through bread and, in doing this, inspire others.

The following ideas are all things that I have done and that people I know have done too.

You may well think of other ways that you can use bread to connect you to others and, as you do this, the likelihood is that you will inspire others to do so too. This is one of the ways revolutions can happen. Step by step, person by person, one loaf at a time. In addition to baking bread for you and your family, you can:

🌿 Give bread as a present. We all have too much stuff. Giving a present that is handmade, nourishing, and will be used rather than creating clutter is always welcome. You can personalize the bread using scoring or by creating dough decorations made from flour and water. Receiving a loaf of bread with your initial on it is a delight. Take homemade bread instead of cakes to fundraising bake sales.

🌿 Find out the whereabouts of your nearest mill that produces stone-ground flour. Support this local business by buying their flour and at the same time optimize the nutritional value and taste of your bread. As well as connecting you to the mill and miller, this can also connect you to the farmer who has grown the grain (sometimes it is the same person).

🌿 See if there are any bakery-based social enterprises or charities operating in your area (local authorities can often help with lists of local organizations). These bakery projects often welcome volunteers.

🌿 Double the amounts to make another full-size loaf or add half again to the original quantities to make a mini loaf alongside your own for someone else. Do you have a relative or neighbor who might appreciate a homemade loaf?

Small loaves are often particularly welcomed by older people whose appetites are not enormous.

- Volunteer to bake bread with children in a local school or with people living in residential care. This is very rewarding and worth jumping through the necessary hoops to do.

- Plan a party (for children or adults) as a bread-baking gathering and each guest can take their loaf home with them.

- Teach someone else—a friend, a child, a grandchild—how to bake bread and spread the love.

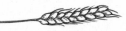

THE LAST CRUST

I started this book with the smell of baking bread wafting through my house, early in the morning, ready for a leisurely weekend or holiday breakfast. This would be a lovely feeling even if it were just me who was to be feasting on that freshly baked bread, but there is something infinitely better about sharing it with others. The instinct to feed, share, and connect with people we know and care about is a strong one. The language of food and of bread is a universal language. Connecting with people who we don't yet know, in our immediate and then wider communities, is also something that can contribute to our satisfaction with life, to our happiness and sense of fulfillment as individuals and to healthy cohesion and mutual understanding in groups. It is what we are built to do. It is the basis of human existence.

This is a self-help book, but helping ourselves is only part of the picture. Self-help is to do with looking after ourselves so that we can be as well as possible—both mentally and physically. It is important to remember, though, that this is not an end in itself, or it shouldn't be. It is a means to an end, and the end is living a full, purposeful life because ultimately what gives us a sense of satisfaction is the feeling of a life well lived. The fulfilled life is one in which we are conscious of our values and the things that really matter to us. Achieving a fulfilled life is helped by having the health and motivation to act and to spend our resources (time and energy, as well as money) in ways that resonate with these beliefs and principles. On our death beds we are unlikely to say that we are glad that we lost 8 pounds on a juice diet when we were 47. On the other hand, we might well be very glad that we looked after our family as best we could, that we worked hard for causes that were important to us, that we had made something original, that we had laughed and had fun with the people we loved, that we had long-lasting friendships, that we contributed to the lives of our communities or the planet, or that we made a difference to others in our private, working, or creative lives.

> The fulfilled life is one in which we are conscious of our values and the things that really matter to us.

Making bread, giving people bread, championing the merits of handmade and real bread, and encouraging others to make bread have contributed to my sense of fulfillment. I fervently hope that it will for you too. Make bread with love and pass it on.

Focaccia

Focaccia is an Italian bread made for sharing. As with so many types of bread, there is plenty of scope for variation and inventiveness. The basic loaf is either rectangular or oval in shape. It is baked in a tray, such as a roasting pan, and is usually about 1 inch deep after baking. This is a bread that works best with white bread flour to give it a good rise. It always has olive oil and sea salt on top, and then you can add what you like. I love the combination of chopped fresh rosemary, black olives, and cherry tomatoes, as the colors are beautiful. You might want to try some chopped chilies, garlic, or red onion. Herbs, such as thyme or basil, are lovely, and grated hard cheese, such as Parmesan, works well too.

A dough scraper will come in really handy for this recipe— if you don't have one you can use a stiff spatula.

Makes 2 focaccia, approximately 13 x 9 x 1 inches each

INGREDIENTS

4¼ cups (18 oz/500 g) white bread flour, plus extra for dusting

2 envelopes (4½ tsp/14 g) fast-acting yeast

2 tsp fine salt (unrefined sea salt if possible)

2 tbsp extra virgin olive oil, plus extra for oiling and drizzling

1⅔ cups (400 ml) warm water

fine semolina flour, for dusting (optional)

flaky sea salt

1 tbsp chopped rosemary leaves

METHOD

1. Start making the focaccia about 3 hours before you want to eat the bread but remember that, for most of this time, the dough will be doing its own thing.

2. Mix the flour, yeast and salt in a large mixing bowl with a wooden spoon.

3. Add the olive oil to the warm water in a measuring cup, then pour most of it (leave about ¼ cup/50 ml in the cup) into the flour mix. Flours differ in how absorbent they are, so you might not need all of the water, but you will need most of it. If there is still dry flour to be incorporated into the dough, add the rest of the water. This should be quite a wet dough.

4. Stir with the spoon until combined and then start to knead the dough in the bowl for about 5 minutes with your hands. It will feel sticky and this is fine; don't be tempted to add any more flour, you can add a little oil to your hands. Try pulling half of the dough to one side and then folding it back on itself, turning the bowl so that you are stretching a different part of the dough as you go around.

5. Lightly oil your work surface with a little olive oil and turn the dough out on to it. This is where a dough scraper can come in handy. They are very good to use with sticky doughs that can end up wrapped around your fingers, as you can use the scraper to clean the dough off your hands so as not to waste it. If you don't have a dough scraper, then you could try to use a stiff silicone or plastic spatula.

6. Now use the scraper or spatula to clean out the mixing bowl. It is worth washing out the mixing bowl now, so you don't get stray lumps of dry dough in your loaf. Dry the bowl and lightly oil it. Oiling the work surface and bowl helps with the stickiness and, for this dough, it is better than adding more flour, which can make the bread too solid.

7. Knead and fold your dough on the work surface again for another 5 minutes, then shape it into a ball and place it back in the oiled bowl. Cover the bowl with a damp dish towel. The cloth should be stretched over the top of the bowl and not touching the dough.

8. Leave the dough in a warm place until it has doubled in size. This will probably take about 1 hour.

9. Pour or scrape (or both) the dough on to the work surface and divide it in half.

10. Line a 13 x 9 x 1-inch baking pan or pans, if you have two, with baking parchment, and sprinkle with flour or fine semolina flour (this is particularly good for stopping sticking and adds a tiny bit of crunch).

11. Put the dough into the pan and then gently push and spread it out until it covers most of the surface. Repeat with a second pan if you have one. If not, put half of the dough back into the bowl, cover it, and put it into a cooler place.

12. Cover the dough in the pan with a damp cloth and leave it to rise for another hour, or until doubled in size again. The dough might rise up to touch the damp cloth, but this doesn't matter, peel the cloth off carefully if it does stick.

13. Heat the oven to 425ºF/220ºC.

14. Your tray or trays of dough should look quite puffy now and you are ready for one of the most satisfying jobs in breadmaking. Drizzle some olive oil over the surface of the dough and then use your fingers to poke holes at

regular intervals all over the surface. If you are lucky, you might have bubbles rising up as you press down and the olive oil will seep into the depressions in a very satisfying way.

15. Now is the point where you can sprinkle the surface with the flaky sea salt (or grated cheese if you are using it) and the rosemary, and add anything else you are using by sticking them into the dough (this is very gratifying too).

16. Take a good look at the beauty of what you have created before putting it all in the oven for approximately 20 minutes. Ovens and doughs vary, but you are aiming for a lightly golden color on top, rather than brown. Focaccia is a bread that can be served warm from the oven.

This hearty bread will create warmth and connection between the lucky people who share it with smiles and laughter and love. Make bread, share love.

Endnote

I began *Bread Therapy* with the hope that, as well as picking up and enjoying reading the book, you would also be inspired to pick up a mixing bowl and flour and get your hands into some dough. Whether you have taken that step yet or not, I hope that you now have a sense of how rich a contribution to your emotional life, as well as to your table, breadmaking can provide.

You will have learned something of how much the experiences you had growing up will have shaped the way you see yourself and your achievements now. I hope that it will also be apparent that however difficult you might have found it to be proud of yourself in the past, it is never too late to develop self-compassion and to learn to accept yourself and what you accomplish with pride and confidence. A paradox at the center of *Bread Therapy* is that it is when we fail—when things go wrong or do not turn out as expected—that we have the best opportunity to practice treating ourselves with the same kindness we would show others. It is in accepting our sometimes imperfect loaves that we can get better at embracing our own limitations. It is in accepting these flaws, seeing ourselves as we are, that we release our potential to blossom.

Learning to be mindful, looking after and nourishing ourselves well, continuing to be curious and creative, understanding our own values, and being true to ourselves will all help us to develop a strong identity and sense of our own worth. It is feeling positive about ourselves that then allows us to grow healthy relationships with others.

I told you how I realized that what mattered to me more than anything else was helping people to know that they are loved. I can think of no better way of showing love to others than by making and giving them real bread that you have made with your own hands. I hope you can feel the love in this book and that you too can bake bread with love and pass it on.

"Shower the people you love with love."
James Taylor

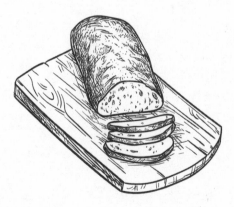

Suggested Reading

Chapter 1
Bertinet, Richard, *Crust*
David, Elizabeth, *English Bread and Yeast Cookery*
Thubten, Gelong, *A Monk's Guide to Happiness*
Whitley, Andrew, *Bread Matters*

Chapter 2
Chatterjee, Rangan, *The 4 Pillar Plan: How to Relax, Eat, Move and Sleep Your Way To a Longer, Healthier Life*
Elliot-Gough, Karl, *The Seven Deadly Whites: Evolution to Devolution— The Rise of the Diseases of Civilization*
Herz, Rachel, *Why You Eat What You Eat*
Pollan, Michael, *Food Rules, An Eater's Manual*
Wilson, Bee, *The Way We Eat Now*
www.beatingeatingdisorders.org.uk for helpful information on eating disorders

Chapter 3
Espe Brown, Edward, *The Tassajara Bread Book*
Csikszentmihalyi, Mihaly, *Flow: The Classic Work on How to Achieve Happiness*
Murdoch, Iris, *The Sovereignty of Good*
Zen Master Dogen and Roshi, Uchiyama Kosho, *How to Cook Your Life: From the Zen Kitchen to Enlightenment*
Sennett, Richard, *The Craftsman*
Whitley, Andrew, *Do Sourdough: Slow Bread for Busy Lives*

Chapter 4

Boxer, Arabella, *First Slice Your Cookbook*
Cameron, Julia, *The Artist's Way*
Lepard, Dan, *The Handmade Loaf*
Wright, Kenneth, *Mirroring and Attunement*

Chapter 5

Eger, Edith, *The Choice*
Frankl, Viktor, E. *Man's Search for Meaning*
Garcia, Hector and Miralles Francesc, *Ikigai: The Japanese Secret to a Long and Happy Life*
Kierkegaard, Soren, *The Sickness unto Death*, translated from the Danish by Alastair Hannay
Perry, Philippa, *The Book You Wish Your Parents Had Read (and Your Children Will Be Glad That You Did)*
Reading, Suzy, *The Little Book of Self-Care*
Yalom, Irvin, *Existential Psychotherapy*

Chapter 6

Bates, Sasha, *Languages of Loss*
Chodron, Pema, *When Things Fall Apart*
Day, Elizabeth, *How to Fail: Everything I've Ever Learned from Things Going Wrong*
Kempton, Beth, *Wabi Sabi: Japanese Wisdom for a Perfectly Imperfect Life*
Navarro, Tomás, *Kintsugi*

Chapter 7

Bottura, Massimo, & Friends, *Bread is Gold: Extraordinary Meals with Ordinary Ingredients*
Buettner, Dan, *The Blue Zones Solution*
Mason, Jane, *Making Bread at Home*
Nilsson, Magnus, *The Nordic Baking Book*
www.realbreadcampaign.org for information on all aspects of real bread and real bakers
www.tcmg.org.uk The Traditional Cornmillers Guild for information about traditional millers in the UK

Glossary

Baking parchment: Paper that stops loaves from sticking to baking sheets. It is also really helpful in lifting your loaves into and out of a Dutch oven. Look for unbleached, compostable parchment. Baking parchment can often be re-used a number of times if it isn't torn or burned. You can buy it as a continuous roll to cut or in fixed lengths.

Baking sheet: A flat, metal pan for baking free-form loaves or buns.

Baking stone: Often called a pizza stone, a thin stone or ceramic slab that is heated in the oven before baking your loaf on it.

Banneton: A basket for proofing your dough. The traditional cane sort leaves a concentric circle pattern on your dough. Some versions have a cloth lining and some are made from wood pulp. I mostly use the cane variety because of the lovely patterns they make on the bread, but the other sorts are equally as good. Bannetons cannot be used for baking, just for proofing.

Bran: The outer layer of whole grains, such as wheat or oats. As well as being rich in fiber, bran contains other nutrients, including B vitamins.

Bread flour: Flour that is made from hard wheat varieties and contains more gluten than all-purpose flour, which allows for well-risen loaves.

Cooling rack: A wire-mesh rack for cooling bread that allows air to circulate under the loaves and stops them getting soggy.

Crumb: The term used for the appearance of the inside of a loaf of bread when you cut it open. It often refers to the pattern and the size of holes in the bread; they can vary from being small and evenly distributed in a dense, whole-grain loaf to large and randomly spread in white sourdough.

Discard: This is the name given to extra or "waste" starter. If you were just to add water and flour without discarding some of the existing starter every time you feed it, then you would end up with too much for the container and the starter would risk being less active. You don't have to throw this excess starter away, though; the discard can be saved in a lidded container in the fridge and can be used to make sourdough crumpets or crackers or added to a yeasted bake another time, though you will be using it to add flavor and to avoid waste—discard will not act as a raising agent. It is hard to find consensus on how long discard can be kept for; I have kept it in a tub in the fridge for a month or more without any problems. As with your main starter, if ever there is any mold growth or unusual smell, then you will need to throw it away.

Dough: The mix of flour, salt, water, and yeast (wild or baker's) that will become bread after rising and baking.

Dough scraper: Also called a bench scraper. A flexible metal or plastic tool for scraping dough from the work surface, mixing bowl, or your hands. They are especially useful for sticky doughs.

Dutch oven: The name for any large lidded casserole (usually cast-iron) which is used as a sort of mini oven inside an ordinary oven. By baking your loaf inside the lidded pot for the first half of the baking time, the steamy atmosphere of a professional bread oven is replicated on a smaller scale. The lid is removed for the second part of the baking to brown the crust.

Emmer: An ancient grain, first grown and eaten in the Bronze and Iron Ages, which is still cultivated and eaten today. The grain, which is related to wheat, produces a creamy- and nutty-flavored flour.

Feeding a starter: Also known as "refreshing a starter," this is the process by which you keep your sourdough starter alive and thriving, particularly before baking with it.

Fermentation: The process before baking, in which the dough develops in volume and taste. There are two processes that make up fermentation in bread. The first is the yeast feeding on the starches or sugars in the dough to produce carbon dioxide and alcohol. The second is the reaction of the flour with water to develop gluten. The second reaction allows for a stretchy structure within the dough to hold little pockets of gas (the alcohol evaporates during baking). The general rule is that the longer the fermentation, the better the taste of the bread.

Folding a dough: This is a variation on kneading. Periodically folding the dough in on itself in a bowl or container during rising will, like kneading, develop and align the gluten strands in the dough. Folding is particularly useful when working with wet doughs that would otherwise stick to your hands too much. A scraper or your fingertips are used to lift one side of the dough and fold it over the rest, the bowl is then turned, and the folding is repeated for each side of the dough. This method is sometimes used during the first rise (or bulk fermentation) of sourdough when the baker might turn and fold the dough every 30 minutes during a 3- or 4-hour period.

Gluten: The general name for the proteins found in many grains, including all varieties of wheat, rye, and barley. There are two main types of protein in flour: gliadin and glutenin. The addition of water to flour forms gluten, which is further developed by kneading and working the dough. Gluten is what gives dough its elasticity and allows it to rise when fermentation occurs during proofing.

Kneading: Sometimes called "working the dough," this process involves using your hands to pull, push, pummel, or stretch your dough and develop its gluten, until the dough becomes smoother and more elastic in texture.

Knocking back: After the dough has risen and usually doubled in size in the first proofing, it needs to have some of the gas already produced pushed out, as this allows the volume, structure, and taste to develop properly in the second rise. To knock the dough back, you give it a gentle, quick knead for a few seconds.

Lame: A specialty tool that is essentially a razor blade in a holder used to score sourdough. It is particularly useful for making elaborate patterns, but a sharp knife will do the trick well for simple scores.

Loaf pan: A deep rectangular pan used to bake a traditionally-shaped sandwich loaf.

Oats: A cereal grain that is whole-grain and prepared in different forms, such as rolled oats, steel-cut oats, oatmeal, and oat flour.

Organic: Organic flour is made from grain that has been grown using farming methods that avoid the use of man-made fertilizers, pesticides, and other additives, or of irradiation or genetic modification.

Oven spring: The expansion of the dough in the oven before the crust forms. This stage is made to last longer during the first part of baking when using a professional oven that produces steam or a Dutch oven. The steam in the oven keeps the skin of the dough soft and therefore allows maximum expansion of the loaf, producing a good oven spring.

Proofing: To proof a dough is to allow it to rise. Dough will rise faster in a warm atmosphere, but is sometimes slowed down or "retarded" deliberately to improve the taste of the bread by being kept in a fridge. Loaves usually require two rises to improve taste, but also to allow the dough to develop enough strength to hold its shape when it is baked. Both under-proofed and over-proofed dough can cause problems for the resultant loaves. Under-proofed loaves will be dense and doughy in the middle; over-proofed loaves will be flat as they have effectively over-inflated and then collapsed.

Real bread: The Real Bread Campaign defines real bread as bread made without the use of additives.

Refreshing a starter: (*see Feeding a starter*)

Rye: Rye flour is made from the berries of a grass plant that grows well in colder climes. It is widely used in northern and eastern Europe. It is lower in gluten than flour made from wheat and therefore produces a denser crumb with smaller bubbles and requires little kneading. Rye dough is also usually made much wetter than other doughs—it can sometimes almost be poured—and is therefore best baked in lined tins.

Scoring: Making a shallow cut or cuts into the upper surface of a loaf to prevent splitting or bursting of the loaf when it is baking and rising in the oven.

Shaping: Shaping takes place before the second rise. Using floured hands, the partially risen dough is turned around while tucking its edges underneath itself. This produces tension in the surface of the dough, which helps the loaf to keep its shape.

Soda bread: A traditional Irish bread that uses baking soda and buttermilk to create a rapid rise; there is no kneading required.

Sourdough: Bread made with only flour, water, and salt. The raising agent is the naturally occurring wild yeasts from the flour and other surfaces. It has a slightly sour flavor and is more digestible for many people.

Spelt: An ancient grain. Bread made with whole-grain spelt flour has a distinctive, nutty flavor. It is a nutritious flour that is naturally high in fiber and contains more protein than wheat.

Starter: The mix of fermented flour and water used to make sourdough bread.

Stone-ground: Flour made from grain ground using millstones. It is nutritionally superior to machine-milled flour, which has had the wheat germ and bran removed.

Unleavened bread: Any bread, usually flatbread, that is made without a raising agent.

Unrefined salt: Unrefined salt comes either from deep salt mines or from sea water through evaporation. It retains the trace minerals that occur in salt's natural state, is not chemically treated, and contains no additives.

Wheat: A grass grown for its seeds, which are ground to make flour. There are many varieties of wheat and it is one of the most widespread cereal crops. Wheat flour is well suited to bread-baking because its gluten content makes for a strong and elastic dough.

Wheat germ: The germ of the wheat is the tiny part of the seed that can germinate to grow into a plant. The germ is rich in polyunsaturated fats.

Whole grain: Intact grains that have not been processed in any way.

Whole-grain flour: Flour made from whole grains that have all of the bran and germ present.

Yeast: A microorganism that converts sugars to alcohol and carbon dioxide, a fermentation process that in turn helps a dough to rise.

Acknowledgments

When I pitched the idea for *Bread Therapy* to Jane Graham-Maw, whom I am so glad to say became my agent, she said three words: "I love it"—these are such glorious words for a writer to hear. From that promising start, Jane has expertly guided me through the process and has championed the book with deftness and decisiveness. *Bread Therapy* ended up in the enthusiastic and skilled hands of my publisher at Yellow Kite, Liz Gough, and the wonderful team at Hodder & Stoughton, including Emma Knight, Grace McCrum, Catriona Horne, Sarah Christie, Niamh Anderson, and Olivia Nightingall. Briony Hartley also worked alongside them and designed these pages so beautifully, with David Wardle designing the cover. The manuscript was passed to my editor, Imogen Fortes, who meticulously shaped the book into the best possible version of itself. I can't tell you what a joy it has been to work with people who get me and my work, and I thank Jane, Liz, and Imogen from the bottom of my heart.

I am lucky enough to have a group of old friends who share my love of food and food writing; they have been unwavering in their faith in me and support for this book. I am indebted to Kristen Frederickson, Sam Goldsmith, Rosie Jones, Orlando Murrin, Katie Socker, and Susan Willis for their unerring affection and encouragement.

My dear friend and comics artist Suzy Varty has also been a creative inspiration and loving support to me for more years than I care to remember—thank you Suzy.

I grew up in the northeast of England. In the eighties and nineties, a trip from Tyneside to the Lake District was not complete without a stop at The Village Bakery at Melmerby. It was run by Andrew Whitley, who led a renaissance in traditional bread-baking. He co-founded The Real Bread Campaign with Sustain and continues the good fight now from Scotland. His earthy, authentic bread was a revelation; the memory of those loaves, and the books he has written to share his knowledge and mission, continue to be an inspiration to me and I thank him for giving me a literal taste and an understanding of what real bread can be.

I can't remember the first loaf of bread I baked myself. I couldn't have known what an important place it would take in my life, but I can be sure it will have been eaten by whichever members of my family were at home. My six darling children, to whom this book is dedicated, are all grown up now, but it still gives me as much pleasure as it ever did to give them good food and, especially, to bake them bread. They have nourished me in return with incredible love and a belief in me that is more precious than anything else in my life. I am full of gratitude to them and to my husband, Tom, who has been my rock throughout. When we first met, Tom insisted he only liked white bread: times have changed and I'm glad to say, so has his taste in bread. Finally, appreciation to my late parents and my brothers and sisters who have always been there for me. Thank you all.